EASY PALEO

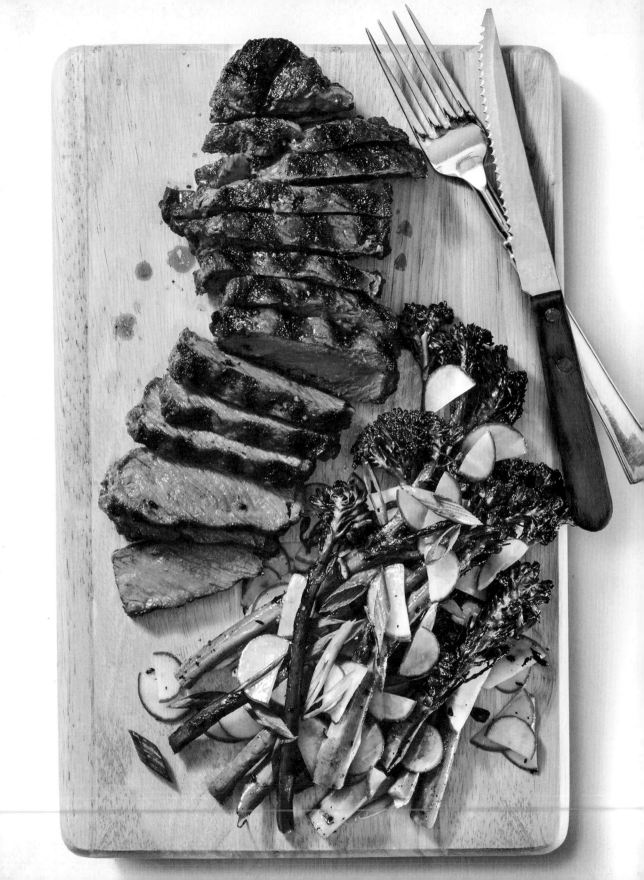

GOOD
HOUSEKEEPING

EASY PALEO

70 DELICIOUS RECIPES

★ GOOD FOOD GUARANTEED ★

HEARST
books

HEARSTBOOKS

An Imprint of Sterling Publishing Co., Inc.
1166 Avenue of the Americas
New York, NY 10036

ISBN 978-1-61837-224-6

The Good Housekeeping Cookbook Seal guarantees that the recipes in this cookbook meet the strict standards
of the Good Housekeeping Research Institute. The Institute has been a source of reliable information and a
consumer advocate since 1900, and established its seal of approval in 1909. Every recipe has been triple-tested
for ease, reliability, and great taste.

Distributed in Canada by Sterling Publishing
c/o Canadian Manda Group, 664 Annette Street
Toronto, Ontario, Canada M6S 2C8
Distributed in the United Kingdom by GMC Distribution Services
Castle Place, 166 High Street, Lewes, East Sussex, England BN7 1XU
Distributed in Australia by NewSouth Books
45 Beach Street, Coogee, NSW 2034, Australia

For information about custom editions, special sales, and premium and corporate purchases,
please contact Sterling Special Sales at 800-805-5489 or specialsales@sterlingpublishing.com.

Manufactured in China

2 4 6 8 10 9 7 5 3 1

www.goodhousekeeping.com
www.sterlingpublishing.com

GOOD HOUSEKEEPING
Jane Francisco
EDITOR IN CHIEF
Melissa Geurts
DESIGN DIRECTOR
Susan Westmoreland
FOOD DIRECTOR
Sharon Franke
KITCHEN APPLIANCES & TECHNOLOGY DIRECTOR
THE GOOD HOUSEKEEPING INSTITUTE

Cover and Interior Design: Phil Buchanan
Project Editor: Carol Prager

CONTENTS

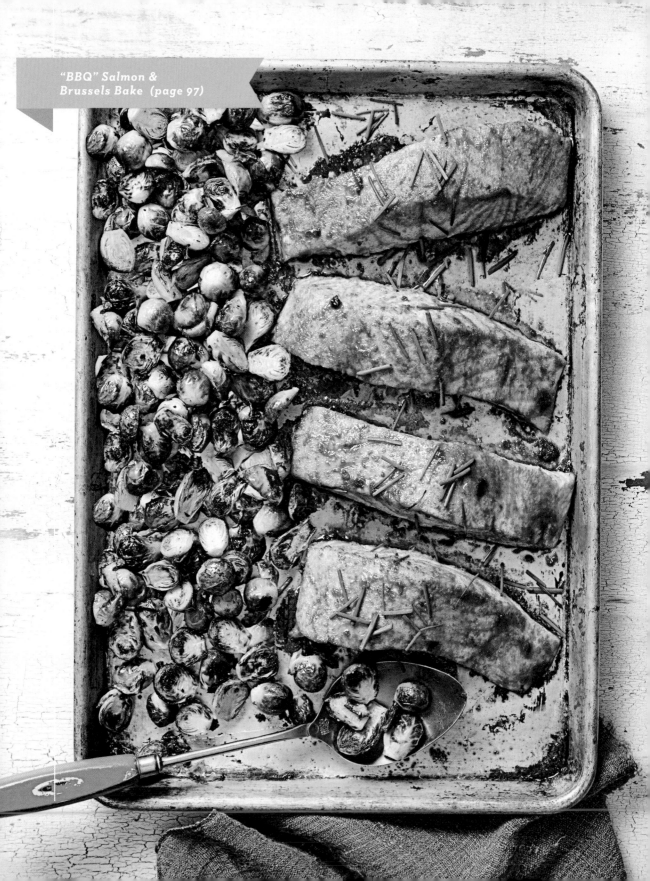

"BBQ" Salmon & Brussels Bake (page 97)

Foreword

Over the past few years, interest in the paleo lifestyle has soared. We are more aware than ever of the benefits of eating healthfully and the problems of not doing so. The paleo diet embraces whole foods and avoids processed foods, wheat and other cereal grains, legumes (including peanuts), dairy, refined sugar, potatoes, salt, and refined vegetable oils.

What's left, you ask? A roster of veggies from avocado to zucchini, lean meat, fish and shellfish, eggs, nuts and seeds, and good-for-you oils like extra virgin olive oil, coconut oil, and nut and seed oils. If you have celiac disease or experience sensitivity to gluten, grains, or legumes, you may unwittingly be following a paleo diet. And if you're looking for a low-carbohydrate diet—which some research has shown is beneficial for weight loss—then the paleo diet's easy guidelines are a good way in.

While *Good Housekeeping* doesn't endorse a strict paleo diet for everyone, we want to provide advice and recipes for those who want to try this plan. *Easy Paleo* gives delicious, veggie-laden, healthful recipes that will keep you satisfied.

So whether you want to dip in and try a few paleo options or streamline your lifestyle, recipes like Caribbean Chicken Thighs, Steak with Argentine Herb Sauce, Ginger-Crusted Salmon with Melon Salsa, and Savory Pumpkin & Sage Soup will convince you that you can be satisfied without grains or dairy. Cavemen never had it so good!

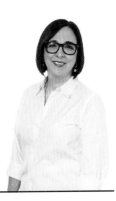

SUSAN WESTMORELAND
Food Director, *Good Housekeeping*

Introduction

If you're looking to limit processed foods in your diet, going paleo makes sense. But if you've hesitated in the past because the plan seems too strict and complicated, *Good Housekeeping Easy Paleo* has everything you need to get started and cook delicious meals. Our take on paleo is surprisingly simple and flexible. From soups and nuts to smart-choice meats and chicken plus plenty of fruits and veggies, it's time to discover a thoroughly modern way of healthy eating.

THE PALEO PRINCIPLE

Follow these three simple rules to eat the paleo way:

1 **THINK OUTSIDE THE "BOX"** (i.e.: can, bottle, or plastic container) and focus on the nutrient-dense foods of our forbearers: fresh fruits and veggies, lean meats, fish, poultry, eggs, healthful oils, and nuts. These pure, whole foods will boost your metabolism naturally.

2 **SKIP PROCESSED FOODS,** cereal grains, legumes (including peanuts), refined sugar, white potatoes, refined oil, and dairy.

3 **TAKE IT EASY ON THE SALT.**

THE PALEO ADVANTAGE

You'll enjoy major health benefits by following our paleo eating plan:

- Lean, healthy proteins (versus carbohydrates) to feel full and satisfied.
- Increasing fresh fruits and veggies to fill your plate.
- Eliminating refined oils (i.e.: canola, corn, peanut, and vegetable oil) in favor of more flavorful, healthful fats.
- Vastly reduce sugar: a vital part of healthy eating according to the USDA, whose current guidelines recommend consuming less than 10 percent of calories per day from added sugars.

ORGANIC VERSUS LOCAL: WHICH IS BETTER?

In the paleo kitchen, it would be best to use ingredients that are both organic and local. However, we are often compelled to choose between the two. The good news is that being aware of where your food comes from and how it's grown makes it easier to decide what type of products to buy. More supermarkets are featuring foods that are both local and organic, plus there are other options you can try:

JOIN A CSA (Community Supported Agriculture). Receive a variety of fresh, organic food from local farmers each week.

SEEK OUT A LOCAL FARMERS' MARKET. Meet the farmers, consume local varieties, and if their products are not organic, ask just how much pesticides they use.

TALK WITH YOUR SMALL, LOCAL FOOD SHOPS. See if they would be willing to request local food varieties from distributors or purchase from regional growers.

THE DRILL ON OIL

Going paleo gives you the opportunity to experiment with a variety of unrefined, super-flavorful oils in your cooking. Choose from the following:

OLIVE OIL/EXTRA-VIRGIN OLIVE OIL

TASTE: Depending on source, from fruity and nutty to herbal and grassy.
BENEFITS: A great source of healthy mono-unsaturated fats, which help control cholesterol levels and have been linked to heart health.

USE: Pure or light olive oil for cooking; extra-virgin olive oil for salads, dressings, and vinaigrettes.

FLAXSEED OIL

TASTE: Clean, crisp, and mildly nutty.
BENEFITS: Contains both omega-3 and omega-6 fatty acids; shown to help increase HDL (good) cholesterol levels.
USE: Highly perishable and extremely sensitive to heat; use only for salad dressings and as a finishing oil.

WALNUT OIL

TASTE: Rich and nutty.
BENEFITS: High in antioxidants and omega-3 fatty acids.
USE: Ideal for salad dressings or brushed onto grilled fish or chicken before serving; avoid heating as the oil can turn slightly bitter.

VIRGIN COCONUT OIL

TASTE: Deep coconut flavor and aroma.
BENEFITS: Rich like butter but dairy- and cholesterol-free; good source of antioxidants.
USE: High-heat cooking like stir-frying; Caribbean and Asian dishes.

AVOCADO OIL

TASTE: Slightly grassy with mild avocado flavor.
BENEFITS: High in vitamin E and omega-3 fatty acids.
USE: Great for roasted, grilled, or sautéed meats and veggies; salsas and salad dressings.

GO NUTS!

A powerhouse of protein and fiber, nuts are a fabulous addition to any paleo recipe—like our Summery Chicken Waldorf Salad (page 42) with walnuts, Salmon Steaks with Tricolor Pepper Relish (page 90) with almonds, or Caramelized Carrots (page 119) with hazelnuts. Nuts are highly perishable, so they need a little TLC. To fully enjoy nuts at their flavorful best, follow these tips for storage and handling:

FRESHNESS TEST Fresh nuts smell mildly nutty and taste sweet. If nuts smell like paint thinner, they're rancid and should be tossed.

CHILLED NUTS Heat causes the fat in nuts to change structure, which creates off odors and flavors. After purchasing, stash nuts in the fridge away from foods with strong odors (i.e.: fish, cabbage, onions), and they'll keep for up to 1 month. Otherwise, freeze them.

STORAGE SMARTS Nuts may be stored in their original sealed packaging. Once opened, transfer nuts to an airtight container to maintain freshness. If you buy nuts in bulk, place in an airtight container in the freezer.

CHOP, CHOP For best flavor, wait to chop nuts until you're ready to use them.

TOASTED = TASTIER NUTS On a jelly-roll pan, spread nuts in a single layer. Bake at 350°F for 8 to 10 minutes or until fragrant. Cool on a wire rack.

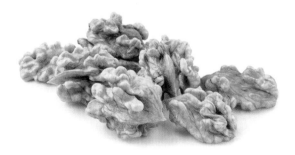

EGGCELLENT EGGS

No way should you deny yourself this protein wonder if you're cooking paleo. Here's what you need to know about the incredible egg and how to cook it right:

CHOOSE CERTIFIED ORGANIC EGGS. These eggs are produced by national USDA standards by hens fed an organic diet (free of conventional pesticides, fungicides, herbicides, or commercial fertilizers).

STORE EGGS PROPERLY. The best place for eggs is in their original carton—not the egg holders on the fridge door. The carton keeps eggs from picking up odors from other foods and also prevents moisture loss. Fresh, refrigerated eggs can last for up to 5 weeks (sometimes longer) and rarely spoil, though they do dry up. If you're worried your eggs are past their prime, crack one in a bowl to give it a sniff test before using—you'll be able to smell a rotten egg immediately.

SEE RED? DON'T WORRY. When a yolk forms, occasionally a blood vessel ruptures, causing a blood spot. These eggs are perfectly safe to eat. You can leave the red dot on the yolk or remove it with the tip of a knife.

Ready to get crackin'? Our basic egg recipes guarantee perfect results every time:

SCRAMBLED EGGS

For each serving, in medium bowl with wire whisk, beat **2 eggs** and **salt** and **pepper to taste** until just blended. In 8-inch skillet, heat **2 teaspoons olive or avocado oil** over medium heat until hot. Add eggs. As eggs begin to set, push egg mixture with heat-safe rubber spatula to form large curds. Continue cooking until eggs have thickened and set.

FRIED EGGS

For each serving, in 8-inch skillet, heat **1 tablespoon olive or avocado oil** over medium heat until hot. Break **2 eggs** into pan; reduce heat to low. For "sunny-side up" eggs, cover and slowly cook until whites are set and yolks have thickened. For "over-easy" eggs, carefully turn eggs over and cook on second side.

POACHED EGGS

In skillet, heat *1½ inches water* to boiling. (For additional flavor, substitute broth, tomato juice, or dry red wine.) Break **cold fresh eggs**, 1 at a time, into cup. Holding cup close to boiling water, slip in eggs. Cook for 3 to 5 minutes or until whites are set and yolks begin to thicken. With slotted spoon, lift out 1 egg and drain, still held in spoon, on paper towels. Repeat with remaining eggs. If desired, trim away any uneven edges of white to give eggs a neater appearance.

COOKED EGGS IN SHELL

Place **eggs** in saucepan with enough *cold water* to cover by at least 1 inch. Heat just to boiling; remove pan from heat and cover. Let eggs stand for 4 to 5 minutes for soft-boiled eggs or 15 minutes for hard-boiled eggs. Carefully pour off water; rinse egg with cold running water to cool and stop the cooking. To peel hard-boiled eggs, gently tap each egg against hard surface until shell is cracked all over. Starting at rounded end, peel egg under cold running water. Unpeeled hard-boiled eggs can be stored in the refrigerator for up to 1 week.

Paleo in the Real World

While there are rules to going paleo, it's not a monolithic way of eating. In fact, as long as you stick to wholesome ingredients, it's okay to diverge from the plan from time to time (so a sprinkle of cheese on a salad or a side of brown rice is okay on occasion). In fact, our recipes feature a number of flexible ingredients. Here are a few of those ingredients (and dishes) that may surprise you:

INGREDIENT	HINT	TRY
Capers	Rinse and drain before using	Cod Livornese (page 94)
Dried Fruits	No sugar added	Lamb & Root Vegetable Tagine (page 62)
Mustard	Preferably with just mustard seeds and vinegar	Citrus Salad (page 28)
Olives	Rinse and drain before using to cut sodium	Chicken with Caramelized Cauliflower & Green Olives (page 76)
Vinegar	Use Champagne, cider, balsamic/white balsamic, red wine, sherry, or white wine vinegar	Watermelon & Crab Gazpacho (page 23)
Wine	Preferably organic without sulfites	Pot Roast with Red Wine Sauce (page 46)

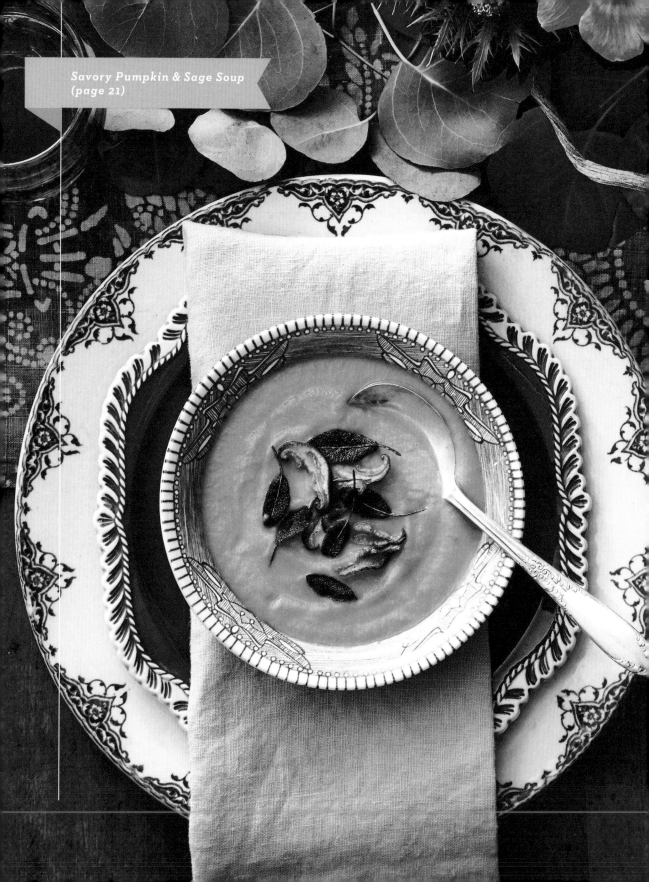

Savory Pumpkin & Sage Soup
(page 21)

1 | Soup's On!

Here's your chance to create a superior bowl of goodness that's chock-full of the freshest fruits and veggies. We've got "souper" recipes to warm you up, like Apple & Parsnip Soup and Savory Pumpkin & Sage Soup. Or keep cool on the hottest summer nights with our no-cook Honeydew & Lime Soup or elegant but easy Watermelon & Crab Gazpacho.

Always using canned broth for soups? If you're serious about going paleo, it's time to break that habit. When it comes to great taste, our homemade Rich Chicken Broth and Rich Vegetable Broth trump the store-bought stuff with a lot less sodium. Equally important, you'll also know exactly what's going in the pot, plus there will be enough extras for other paleo meals. Best of all, since the onions don't need peeling and a rough cut is perfectly acceptable for the veggies, prep takes minutes—not hours.

Rich Chicken
BROTH

Our DIY chicken broth is easier than you think—plus, you probably have all the ingredients in the pantry or fridge. Another bonus? The cooked chicken can be used in other recipes.

ACTIVE TIME: 10 MINUTES   **TOTAL TIME:** 4 HOURS 40 MINUTES PLUS COOLING
MAKES: ABOUT 5 CUPS

1   chicken (3 to 3½ pounds), including neck (giblets reserved for another use)

2   carrots, cut into 2-inch pieces

1   stalk celery, cut into 2-inch pieces

1   medium onion, cut into quarters

5   fresh parsley sprigs

1   garlic clove

½   teaspoon dried thyme

½   bay leaf

1   teaspoon salt

1 In 6-quart saucepot, combine chicken, chicken neck, carrots, celery, onion, parsley, garlic, thyme, bay leaf, and *3 quarts water* or enough *water to cover*; heat to boiling over high heat. Skim foam from surface. Reduce heat and simmer for 1 hour, turning chicken once and skimming.

2 Remove from heat; transfer chicken to large bowl. When cool enough to handle, remove skin and bones from chicken. (Reserve chicken for another use.) Return skin and bones to pot and heat to boiling. Skim foam; reduce heat and simmer for 3 hours.

3 Strain broth through colander into large bowl; discard solids and stir in salt. Strain again through sieve into containers; cool. Cover and refrigerate to use within 3 days, or freeze for up to 4 months.

4 To use, skim fat from surface of broth and discard.

....

EACH 1-CUP SERVING: ABOUT 35 CALORIES, 3G PROTEIN, 4G CARBOHYDRATE, 1G TOTAL FAT (1G SATURATED), 0G FIBER, 3MG CHOLESTEROL, 91MG SODIUM.

Pressure Cooker
CHICKEN BROTH

Prepare Rich Chicken Broth as directed, but in step 1, use 6-quart pressure cooker and only *4 cups water*. Following manufacturer's directions, cover pressure cooker and bring up to high pressure (15 pounds). Cook for 15 minutes. Remove cooker from heat, allow pressure to drop for 5 minutes, and then follow manufacturer's directions for quick release of pressure.

Liquid Gold

Here are the essentials you'll need to make the ultimate chicken broth.

GO COLD. Starting with cold water allows the impurities from the chicken bones to collect on top of the water, like foam. Just skim it off with a spoon.

COOK LOW AND SLOW. Once the broth comes to a boil, reduce the heat and simmer (only a few bubbles should hit the surface). Boiling turns chicken broth cloudy.

LOSE THE LID. Simmer chicken broth uncovered so it can reduce in volume, allowing the flavors to concentrate.

SKIM THE FAT. After chicken broth cools, remove any solidified fat from the surface with a slotted spoon.

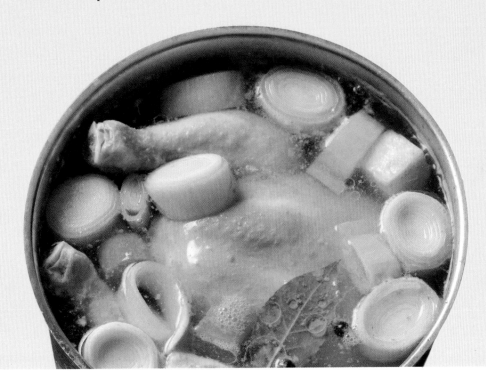

Rich Vegetable
BROTH

We use six kinds of veggies in this exceptional both.
For an Asian twist, add minced lemongrass, minced fresh ginger,
or chopped fresh cilantro during the last 15 minutes of cooking.

ACTIVE TIME: 25 MINUTES **TOTAL TIME:** 2 HOURS 25 MINUTES PLUS COOLING
MAKES: ABOUT 6 CUPS

4   large leeks

2 to 4 garlic cloves, not peeled

Salt

2   fennel bulbs, trimmed and chopped

6   parsnips, peeled and thinly sliced

4   large carrots, thinly sliced

4   stalks celery with leaves, thinly sliced

4   ounces mushrooms, trimmed and thinly sliced

10 fresh parsley sprigs

4   fresh thyme sprigs

2   bay leaves

1   teaspoon whole black peppercorns

Ground black pepper

1 Cut off roots and trim dark green tops from leeks; thinly slice leeks. Rinse leeks thoroughly in large bowl of *cold water*, swishing to remove sand; transfer to colander to drain, leaving sand in bottom of bowl.

2 In 6-quart saucepot, combine leeks, garlic, *1 cup water*, and pinch salt; heat to boiling over high heat. Reduce heat to medium; cover and cook until leeks are tender, about 15 minutes.

3 Add fennel, parsnips, carrots, celery, mushrooms, parsley, thyme, bay leaves, peppercorns, and *12 cups water*. Heat to boiling over high heat; reduce heat and simmer, uncovered, for at least 1½ hours.

4 Taste and continue cooking if flavor is not concentrated enough. Stir in 1 teaspoon salt and pepper to taste. Strain broth through fine mesh sieve into containers, pressing on solids with back of wooden spoon to extract liquid; cool. Cover and refrigerate to use within 3 days, or freeze for up to 4 months.

EACH SERVING: ABOUT 11 CALORIES, 0G PROTEIN, 2G CARBOHYDRATE, 0G TOTAL FAT, 0G FIBER, 0MG CHOLESTEROL, 358MG SODIUM.

Use Your Scraps

Jazz up our Rich Vegetable Broth (at left) or Rich Chicken Broth (page 14) by adding the trimmings from your favorite seasonal veggies. Save any roots, stalks, stems, ends, and peelings during the week. Wash and chop each batch into similar sizes and stash in an airtight bag or container in the fridge (if you're collecting for longer than one week, freeze them). Here are our veggie picks for each season:

WINTER
Kale

Swiss chard

Onions

SUMMER
Zucchini

Green beans

Golden beets

SPRING
Green onions

Asparagus

Lettuce

FALL
Eggplant

Butternut squash

Tomatoes

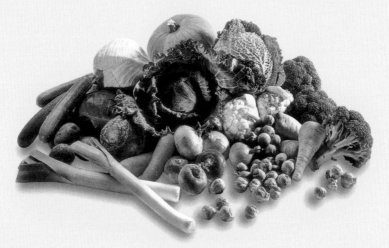

NOTE: Avoid cabbage, Brussels sprouts, broccoli, cauliflower, turnips, rutabagas, and artichokes. Their flavors will overpower your broth.

NOT YOUR GRANDMA'S
Vegetable Soup

Beets give this hearty soup its vibrant red hue.
While available year-round, beets are at their
flavorful best in late summer and autumn.

ACTIVE TIME: 15 MINUTES   **TOTAL TIME:** 1 HOUR 15 MINUTES
MAKES: 5 MAIN-DISH SERVINGS

1 tablespoon olive oil

1 medium onion, chopped

1 garlic clove, crushed with press

½ teaspoon ground allspice

1 can (14½ ounces) diced tomatoes

1 pound beets (not including tops)

6 cups sliced green cabbage (1 pound)

3 large carrots, cut into ½-inch chunks

1¾ cups Rich Vegetable Broth (page 16) or 1 can
   (14½ ounces) lower-sodium vegetable broth

1 bay leaf

¾ teaspoon salt

2 tablespoons red wine vinegar

¼ cup loosely packed fresh dill or parsley,
   chopped

1 In 5- to 6-quart saucepot, heat oil over
medium heat until hot. Add onion and cook,
stirring occasionally, for about 8 minutes or until
tender. Stir in garlic and allspice; cook for 30
seconds. Add tomatoes and cook for 5 minutes.

2 Meanwhile, peel beets and shred in food
processor (or on coarse side of box grater).

3 Into saucepot with onion mixture, stir beets,
cabbage, carrots, *4 cups water*, broth, bay leaf,
and salt; heat to boiling over high heat.

4 Reduce heat to medium-low; cover and simmer
for about 30 minutes or until all vegetables are
tender. Remove bay leaf. Stir in vinegar and dill.

EACH SERVING: ABOUT 160 CALORIES, 5G PROTEIN,
27G CARBOHYDRATE, 5G TOTAL FAT (1G SATURATED),
6G FIBER, 5MG CHOLESTEROL, 920MG SODIUM.

TIP

Always wear rubber gloves while peeling
beets to avoid getting red all over your
hands. Any kind will do: The juice washes
right off. For easy cleanup, peel beets in
the sink.

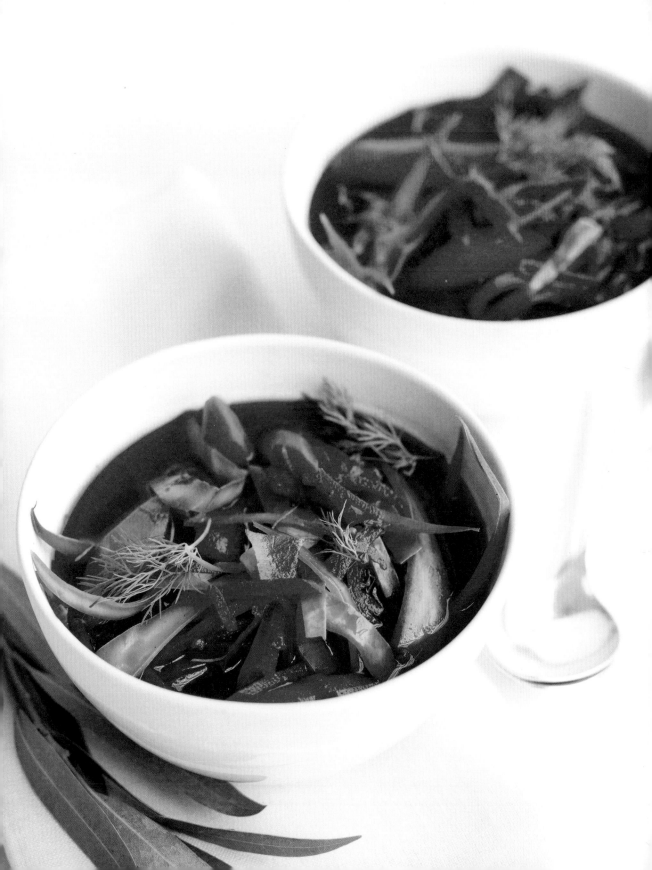

Apple & Parsnip
SOUP

Apples add a touch of sweetness to this soothing pureed soup.
It's equally delicious with our Rich Vegetable Broth (page 16).

ACTIVE TIME: 15 MINUTES   **TOTAL TIME:** 35 MINUTES
MAKES: 6 FIRST-COURSE SERVINGS (ABOUT 9 CUPS)

4 cups Rich Chicken Broth (page 14) or 1 package (32 ounces) lower-sodium chicken broth

1 tablespoon olive oil

2 large shallots, finely chopped (½ cup)

1 stalk celery, finely chopped

2 pounds McIntosh or Braeburn apples (4 to 6 medium), peeled and chopped

1 pound parsnips, peeled and chopped

¼ teaspoon dried thyme

½ teaspoon salt

¼ teaspoon ground black pepper

Roasted, hulled pumpkin seeds, for garnish

1 In covered 2-quart saucepan, heat chicken broth and *2 cups water* to boiling over high heat.

2 Meanwhile, in 5- to 6-quart saucepot, heat oil over medium heat until hot. Add shallots and celery and cook, stirring occasionally, for about 5 minutes or until softened and lightly browned. Add apples, parsnips, thyme, salt, and pepper; cook, stirring, for 1 minute.

3 Add hot broth mixture to saucepot; cover and heat to boiling over high heat. Reduce heat to low; cover and simmer for 6 to 7 minutes or until parsnips are very tender.

4 Spoon one-third of apple mixture into blender; cover, with center part of cover removed to let steam escape, and puree until smooth. Pour puree into bowl. Repeat with remaining mixture. Return to saucepot to reheat. Garnish with pumpkin seeds to serve.

EACH SERVING: ABOUT 160 CALORIES, 3G PROTEIN, 34G CARBOHYDRATE, 3G TOTAL FAT (0G SATURATED), 6G FIBER, 0MG CHOLESTEROL, 600MG SODIUM.

TIP

If you have an immersion blender, use it to puree the soup right in the pot.

Savory Pumpkin & Sage
SOUP

This festive soup with an elegant sage and mushroom garnish
is perfect for entertaining. For photo, see page 12.

ACTIVE TIME: 25 MINUTES   **TOTAL TIME:** 1 HOUR 30 MINUTES
MAKES: 8 FIRST-COURSE SERVINGS (ABOUT 10 CUPS)

¼ cup olive oil

3 large sweet onions, sliced

1¼ teaspoons salt

3 garlic cloves, chopped

2 large fresh sage leaves, chopped

2 teaspoons grated, peeled fresh ginger

¼ teaspoon ground nutmeg

8 cups Rich Vegetable (page 16) or Rich Chicken
   (page 14) Broth or 2 cartons (32 ounces each)
   lower-sodium vegetable or chicken broth

3 cans (15 ounces each) pure pumpkin

1 tablespoon fresh lemon juice

¼ teaspoon ground black pepper

SAGE & SHIITAKE GARNISH

Olive oil

24 small fresh sage leaves

2 packages (3½ ounces each) shiitake
   mushrooms, stemmed and very thinly sliced

Salt

1 In 5-quart saucepot, heat oil over medium heat
until hot. Add onions and ¼ teaspoon salt; cook,
stirring occasionally, for 40 minutes or until
deep golden brown. Add garlic, sage, ginger, and
nutmeg; cook, stirring occasionally, for 5 minutes
or until garlic is golden. Add broth and pumpkin.
Heat to simmering over high heat, stirring until
browned bits are loosened from bottom of pan.
Reduce heat to maintain simmer; cook, stirring
occasionally, for 20 minutes.

2 With immersion blender or in batches in
blender, puree soup until smooth. Stir in lemon
juice, remaining 1 teaspoon salt, and pepper.

3 **Prepare Sage & Shiitake Garnish:** Meanwhile,
in 2-quart saucepan, heat 1 inch olive oil over high
heat until hot but not smoking. Add sage leaves and
fry, stirring occasionally, for 1 to 2 minutes or until
leaves are browned. With slotted spoon, transfer to
large paper towel-lined plate; sprinkle with pinch salt.
In batches, add mushrooms to hot oil. Fry, stirring
occasionally, for 2 minutes or until deep golden
brown. Transfer to same plate as sage; sprinkle with
pinch salt. Cool completely. Garnish can be made up
to 3 hours ahead. Let stand at room temperature.

EACH SERVING: ABOUT 215 CALORIES, 5G PROTEIN,
32G CARBOHYDRATE, 10G TOTAL FAT (1G SATURATED),
9G FIBER, 0MG CHOLESTEROL, 750MG SODIUM.

TIP
This recipe can be prepared and chilled
for up to 2 days. Reheat over medium heat.
If the soup is too thick, add water or broth
to reach desired consistency.

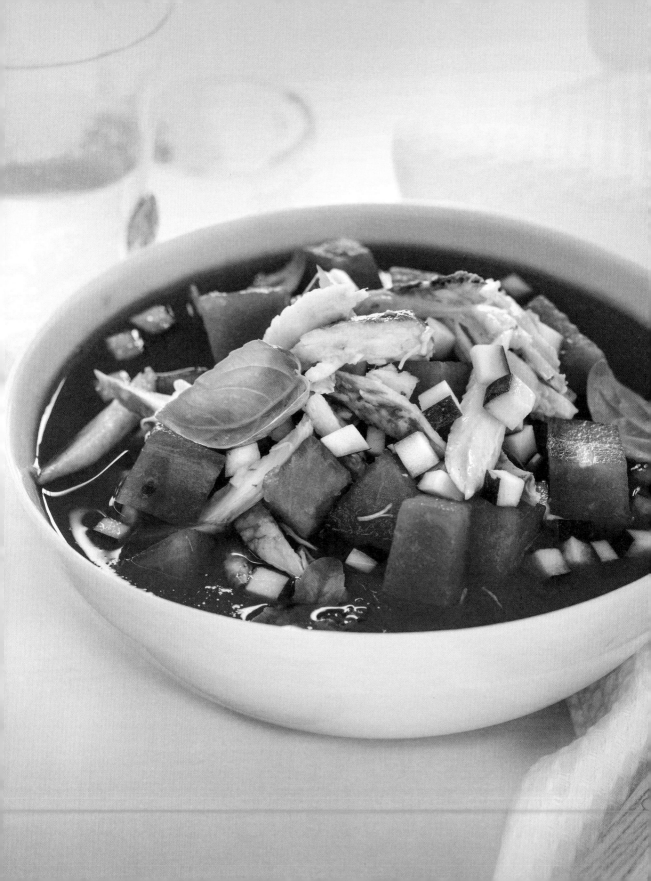

Watermelon & Crab
GAZPACHO

Tomatoes are a fruit, so it's not so radical that
we paired summer's best with juicy watermelon.
The addition of crabmeat makes this soup a satisfying main dish.

TOTAL TIME: 25 MINUTES PLUS CHILLING   **MAKES:** 4 MAIN-DISH SERVINGS

- 2   pounds ripe tomatoes, cut in quarters
- ¼   cup packed fresh basil leaves, plus additional for garnish
- ¼   cup red wine vinegar
- 5   cups seedless watermelon cubes (from 3-pound piece of watermelon with rind)
- 2   small garlic cloves, peeled
- ⅓   cup plus 1 tablespoon extra-virgin olive oil
- ½   teaspoon salt
- ¼   teaspoon ground black pepper
- 1   zucchini (4 ounces), finely chopped
- 1   cup lump crabmeat, picked over

1 In food processor with knife blade attached, pulse tomatoes, basil leaves, vinegar, 4 cups watermelon cubes, 1 garlic clove, ⅓ cup oil, salt, and pepper until pureed.

2 Set medium-mesh sieve over medium bowl. Pour watermelon mixture through sieve, pressing on solids to extract all liquid; discard solids. Cover and refrigerate until chilled, at least 4 hours or up to overnight. Place chopped zucchini and remaining 1 cup watermelon in another bowl; cover and refrigerate overnight.

3 Divide soup among four serving bowls. Top evenly with zucchini, watermelon, and crab. Garnish with basil leaves.

EACH SERVING: ABOUT 321 CALORIES, 8G PROTEIN, 26G CARBOHYDRATE, 23G TOTAL FAT (3G SATURATED), 3G FIBER, 29MG CHOLESTEROL, 382MG SODIUM.

TIP

Buy fresh or frozen crabmeat if available, as it's more flavorful than canned. We prefer lump crabmeat, as it contains the largest chunks.

Honeydew & Lime
SOUP

The gentle sweetness of honeydew melon creates the perfect base
for this refreshing, cold summer soup.

TOTAL TIME: 10 MINUTES PLUS CHILLING   **MAKES:** 6 FIRST-COURSE SERVINGS

1   honeydew melon (5 pounds), chilled
    and cut into 1-inch chunks

¼   cup fresh lime juice

¼   cup loosely packed fresh cilantro leaves

1   teaspoon jalapeño hot sauce

⅛   teaspoon salt

In blender, pulse melon with lime juice, cilantro, hot sauce, and salt until pureed. Transfer soup to large bowl or pitcher; cover and refrigerate for at least 2 hours or until chilled. Stir before serving.

EACH SERVING: ABOUT 85 CALORIES, 1G PROTEIN, 23G CARBOHYDRATE, 0G TOTAL FAT, 2G FIBER, 0MG CHOLESTEROL, 80MG SODIUM.

TIP

This recipe is also terrific with a variety of melons, like cantaloupe, Crenshaw, or casaba melon.

Sweet Beet
SOUP

This soup can be prepped in just minutes thanks to minimally processed, precooked beets. You'll find them refrigerated in the produce section of the supermarket.

ACTIVE TIME: 15 MINUTES **TOTAL TIME:** 25 MINUTES PLUS CHILLING
MAKES: 4 FIRST-COURSE SERVINGS (ABOUT 5 CUPS)

1 tablespoon olive oil

1 medium onion, thinly sliced

½ teaspoon salt

2 packages (8.8 ounces each) cooked, refrigerated beets

1 Granny Smith apple, peeled and chopped

2 cups Rich Vegetable (page 16) or Rich Chicken (page 14) Broth, or lower-sodium vegetable or chicken broth

Fresh dill sprigs, for garnish

1 In 10-inch skillet, heat oil over medium-high heat until hot. Add onion and pinch salt. Cook, stirring frequently, for about 5 minutes or until browned and starting to soften. Let cool.

2 In blender, puree onion mixture, beets, apple, broth, and salt until smooth. Refrigerate until chilled, at least 3 hours or up to overnight.

3 To serve, garnish with dill.

. . . .

EACH SERVING: ABOUT 121 CALORIES, 3G PROTEIN, 24G CARBOHYDRATE, 4G TOTAL FAT (1G SATURATED), 4G FIBER, 0MG CHOLESTEROL, 551MG SODIUM.

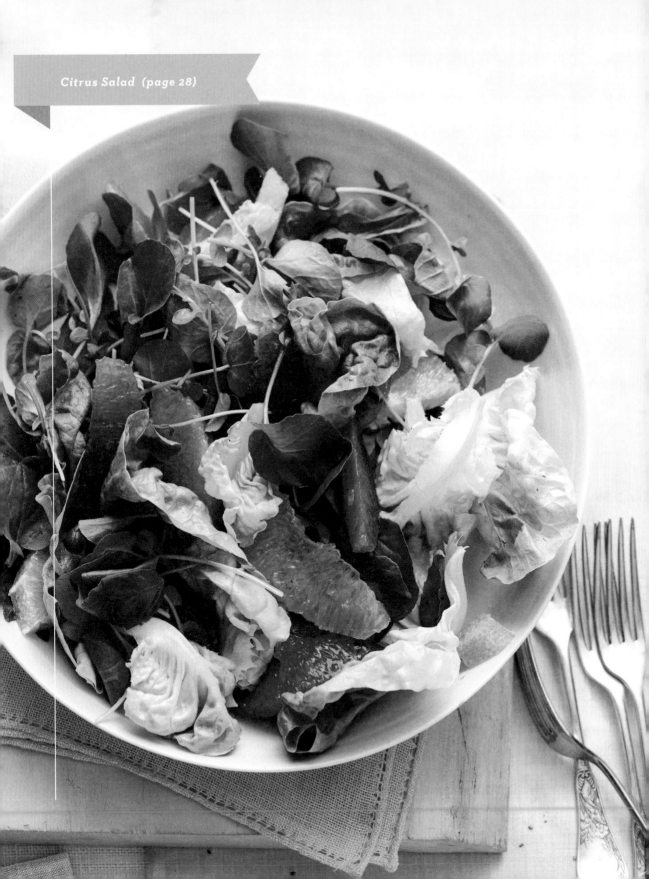

Citrus Salad (page 28)

2 | Big Sides, Big Salads

We've got the perfect paleo salad for any occasion. Choose from our hearty main dish recipes like Summery Chicken Waldorf Salad or Balsamic Roast Pork with Berry Salad. Pair your favorite meat, poultry, or seafood recipe with a simple side like our Radish & Arugula Salad. Or toss up a big batch salad for a crowd, like our Jicama & Orange Salad or Cucumber-Pomegranate Salad. You can even create your own salads, thanks to our guide to greens and trio of paleo-friendly dressings.

Citrus
SALAD

This gorgeous salad with orange, grapefruit, and lemon dressing is perfect for company, as it can be prepped up to 3 days ahead. For photo, see page 26.

TOTAL TIME: 25 MINUTES PLUS CHILLING **MAKES:** 6 SIDE-DISH SERVINGS

2 navel oranges

2 red or pink grapefruits

2 tablespoons fresh lemon juice

1 tablespoon white wine vinegar

2 teaspoons Dijon mustard

¼ teaspoon salt

¼ teaspoon ground black pepper

3 tablespoons extra-virgin olive or avocado oil

1 bunch upland cress or watercress (3 ounces), trimmed

1 head Boston lettuce, torn

¼ cup packed fresh basil leaves, torn if large

1 Cut peel and white pith off oranges. Cut on either side of membranes to remove each section from oranges; place in medium bowl. Repeat with grapefruits, placing in same bowl. Sections can be covered and refrigerated for up to 3 days.

2 In small bowl with wire whisk, mix lemon juice, vinegar, mustard, salt, and black pepper until well blended. In thin steady stream, whisk in oil until well blended. Dressing can be covered and refrigerated for up to 3 days; whisk well before using.

3 In large bowl, gently toss cress, lettuce, and basil with dressing until well coated. Top with citrus sections.

EACH SERVING: ABOUT 125 CALORIES, 2G PROTEIN, 16G CARBOHYDRATE, 7G TOTAL FAT (1G SATURATED), 2G FIBER, 0MG CHOLESTEROL, 145MG SODIUM.

TIP

Look for upland cress at the farmers' market in the spring. The petite leaves have a mild flavor, lingering sharpness, and delicate, peppery taste.

Jicama & Orange
SALAD

This refreshing salad, with in-season jicama and navel oranges,
will brighten up any winter meal.

TOTAL TIME: 35 MINUTES   **MAKES:** 10 SIDE-DISH SERVINGS

1   jicama (1 pound)

½   English (seedless) cucumber

2   medium navel oranges

2   limes

½   cup packed fresh cilantro leaves, coarsely
     chopped

1½   teaspoons olive oil

Pinch cayenne (ground red) pepper

⅛   teaspoon salt

1   Using sharp knife, trim top and bottom of jicama and generously peel tough brown skin. Cut jicama into matchstick-size pieces; you should have about 4 cups. Peel cucumber in alternating strips; cut in half lengthwise, then into ¼-inch-thick half-moons.

2   With knife, cut peel and white pith from oranges and discard. Cut each orange crosswise into ¼-inch rounds; cut each round in half and transfer to large bowl. From limes, grate 1 teaspoon peel and squeeze 2½ tablespoons juice.

3   To bowl with oranges, add jicama, cucumber, lime peel and juice, cilantro, oil, cayenne, and salt; toss well. Serve immediately or refrigerate for up to 4 hours.

EACH SERVING: ABOUT 40 CALORIES, 1G PROTEIN, 8G CARBOHYDRATE, 1G TOTAL FAT (0G SATURATED), 3G FIBER, 0MG CHOLESTEROL, 35MG SODIUM.

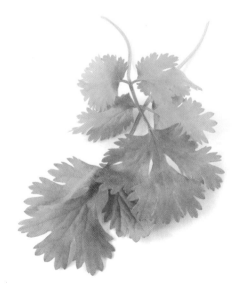

TIP

To test if a jicama is super fresh, scratch the skin; it should be thin, with the creamy flesh juicy underneath.

Cucumber-Pomegranate
SALAD

Sweet-tart pomegranate, a member of the berry
family, is rich in potassium and vitamin C.
It's also a great source of fiber.

TOTAL TIME: 30 MINUTES **MAKES:** 12 SIDE-DISH SERVINGS

1 lemon

⅓ cup extra-virgin olive oil

3 tablespoons Champagne vinegar

½ teaspoon salt

½ teaspoon ground black pepper

1½ pounds fennel bulbs (4 small or 2 large)

1 English seedless cucumber

1 Granny Smith apple, halved and very
thinly sliced

½ cup fresh pomegranate seeds
(from 1 pomegranate)

1 From lemon, grate ½ teaspoon peel and squeeze
2 tablespoons juice. In medium bowl with wire
whisk, mix oil, vinegar, lemon peel and juice,
¼ teaspoon salt, and pepper until well blended.
Dressing can be refrigerated for up to 2 days.

2 Pluck 2 tablespoons fennel fronds from fennel
tops and reserve for garnish. Trim and core fennel.
With adjustable-blade slicer or very sharp knife,
very thinly slice fennel. With vegetable peeler, peel
alternating strips from cucumber skin, then thinly
slice cucumber crosswise at an angle.

3 On large serving platter, layer fennel, cucumber,
and apple. Whisk dressing again and drizzle all
over. Top salad with pomegranate seeds and
garnish with fennel fronds. Sprinkle remaining
¼ teaspoon salt all over.

EACH SERVING: ABOUT 85 CALORIES, 1G PROTEIN,
8G CARBOHYDRATE, 6G TOTAL FAT (1G SATURATED),
2G FIBER, 0MG CHOLESTEROL, 120MG SODIUM.

TIP

If you can only find fennel bulbs without
their tops, substitute 2 tablespoons small
fresh dill sprigs.

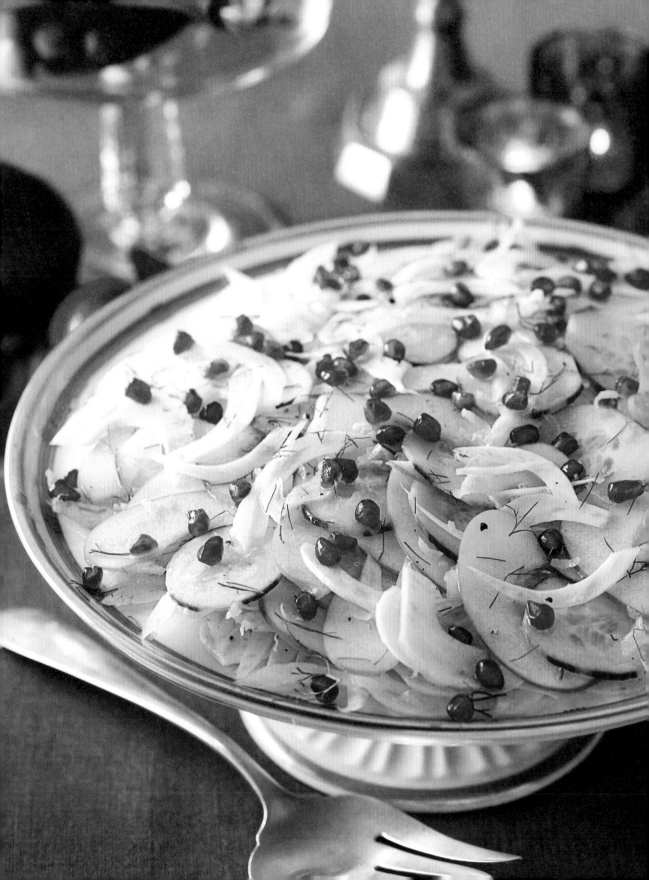

Radish & Arugula
SALAD

This springtime salad has plenty of crunch,
thanks to peppery-sweet radishes and roasted almonds.

TOTAL TIME: 20 MINUTES   **MAKES:** 6 SIDE-DISH SERVINGS

1 medium carrot, peeled

3 tablespoons extra-virgin olive or avocado oil

1 tablespoon fresh lemon juice

1 tablespoon red wine vinegar

¼ teaspoon salt

⅛ teaspoon ground black pepper

4 small heads Belgian endive, trimmed and thinly sliced on an angle

8 ounces radishes, trimmed and cut into quarters

2 cups baby or wild arugula

¼ cup roasted salted almonds, chopped

1 With vegetable peeler, peel carrot into ribbons.

2 In large bowl with wire whisk, mix oil, lemon juice, vinegar, salt, and pepper until well blended. Add endive, radishes, arugula, carrot ribbons, and almonds; toss until combined.

EACH SERVING: ABOUT 115 CALORIES, 2G PROTEIN, 5G CARBOHYDRATE, 10G TOTAL FAT (1G SATURATED), 3G FIBER, 0MG CHOLESTEROL, 140MG SODIUM.

TIP

When shopping for radishes, buy them with their leafy green tops (they're the freshest). Save the greens—they're delicious when sautéed and served with scrambled eggs.

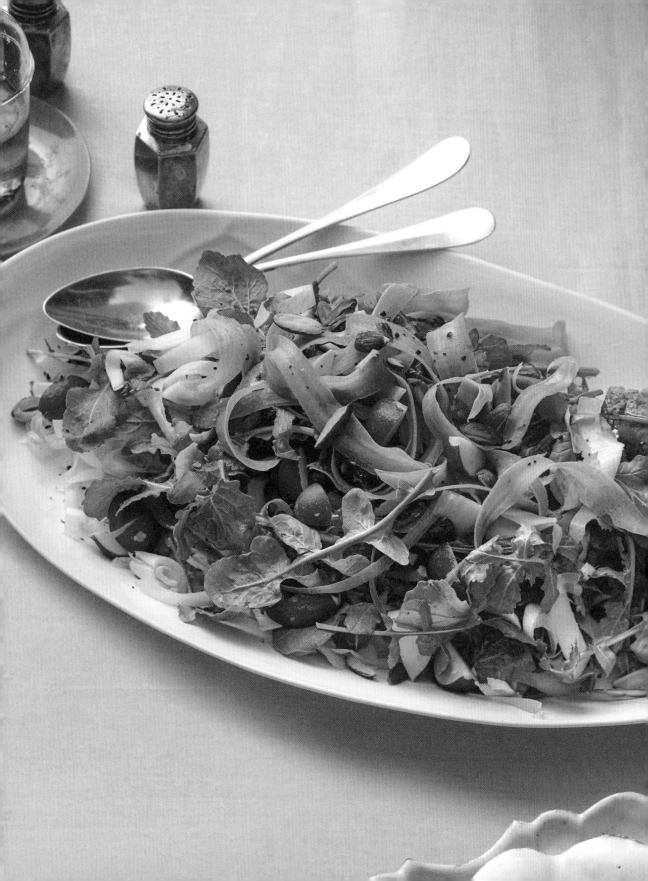

A Mixed Bag

What do our Grilled Watermelon & Peach Salad (page 36), Shrimp with Grilled Nectarines (page 39), and Summery Chicken Waldorf Salad (page 42) have in common? All feature mixed salad greens (sometimes called spring salad mix). Often a combo of tender baby lettuces, the variety of greens can vary from brand to brand. These are some of our favorites:

OAKLEAF

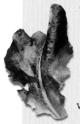

Tender red- or green-hued leaves with a similar shape to that of an oak tree (hence its name). Mild and delicate-tasting, oakleaf makes a great bed for food and won't compete with other flavors.

TATSOI

An Asian green with small, rounded leaves and a mild, mustard-like flavor. Its texture is similar to baby spinach.

MIZUNA

A Japanese mustard green with small jagged edges that adds great texture to salads. Relatively pungent-tasting, it still mixes well with other lettuces.

FRISÉE

(AKA: CURLY ENDIVE, CHICORY, CHICORY ENDIVE, CURLY CHICORY)

These curled leaves tinged with yellow and green are slightly bitter in taste. The crunchy stems make a nice counterpart to soft baby lettuces.

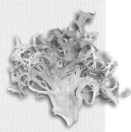

LOLLO ROSSO

Tender and mildly flavored, this lettuce of Italian heritage is distinguished by its deep-red, ruffled leaves.

TIP

Concoct your own mix of greens from the farmers' market! Calculate 3 ounces per 2 cups of salad mix.

All Dressed Up

Want more paleo salads? First step, lose those bottled dressings
with the laundry list of additives. Next, choose a zingy
paleo dressing (below), and toss. Done!

CLASSIC SALAD DRESSING

In medium bowl with wire whisk, mix **¼ cup red wine vinegar**, **1 tablespoon Dijon mustard**, **¼ teaspoon salt**, and **¼ teaspoon ground black pepper**. In thin steady stream, whisk in **½ cup extra-virgin olive**, **avocado**, **or flaxseed oil** until well blended. Cover and refrigerate for up to 3 days. Makes ¾ cup.

EACH 2-TABLESPOON SERVING: ABOUT 165 CALORIES, 0G PROTEIN, 0G CARBOHYDRATE, 18G TOTAL FAT (2G SATURATED), 0G FIBER, 0MG CHOLESTEROL, 110MG SODIUM.

LEMON-OREGANO DRESSING

In medium bowl with wire whisk, mix **⅓ cup fresh lemon juice**; **1 teaspoon Dijon mustard**; **½ teaspoon dried oregano**; **½ small garlic clove**, crushed with press; **¼ teaspoon salt**; and **¼ teaspoon ground black pepper**. In thin steady stream, whisk in **⅓ cup extra-virgin olive or avocado oil** until well blended. Cover and refrigerate up to overnight. Makes ⅔ cup.

EACH 2-TABLESPOON SERVING: ABOUT 120 CALORIES, 0G PROTEIN, 2G CARBOHYDRATE, 13G TOTAL FAT (2G SATURATED), 0G FIBER, 0MG CHOLESTEROL, 110MG SODIUM.

CILANTRO-LIME DRESSING

Prepare outdoor grill for direct grilling over medium heat. Place **1 small poblano pepper** on hot grill rack. Cook for 12 to 15 minutes or until blackened all over, turning occasionally. Wrap pepper in foil; let cool. Remove pepper from foil; peel off skin and discard. Remove and discard stem and seeds. In blender or food processor with knife blade attached, puree pepper, **20 sprigs fresh cilantro**, **½ cup fresh lime juice**, **¼ teaspoon salt**, and **¼ teaspoon ground black pepper** until smooth. With blender running, gradually add **¼ cup olive or avocado oil** until blended. Makes 1 cup.

EACH 2-TABLESPOON SERVING: ABOUT 70 CALORIES, 0G PROTEIN, 2G CARBOHYDRATE, 7G TOTAL FAT (1G SATURATED), 0G FIBER, 0MG CHOLESTEROL, 75MG SODIUM.

Grilled Watermelon & Peach
SALAD

Grill summer fruit at its peak and you'll need
little embellishment, like this sensational
recipe with mixed greens and sherry vinaigrette.

ACTIVE TIME: 10 MINUTES **TOTAL TIME:** 20 MINUTES
MAKES: 4 SIDE-DISH SERVINGS

4 peaches, halved and pitted

8 wedges watermelon, each ½-inch thick

1 container (5 ounces) mixed salad greens

2 tablespoons olive or avocado oil

1 tablespoon sherry vinegar

½ teaspoon salt

½ teaspoon ground black pepper

1 Prepare outdoor grill for direct grilling over medium heat.

2 Brush cut sides of peaches with oil; place on hot grill rack. Cook for 6 to 8 minutes or until grill marks appear and peaches soften slightly, turning over once.

3 Pat watermelon dry; place on hot grill rack. Cook for 3 to 4 minutes or until grill marks appear, turning over once.

4 Arrange greens on large platter. Top with watermelon and peaches; drizzle with oil and vinegar and sprinkle with salt and pepper.

EACH SERVING: ABOUT 166 CALORIES, 2G PROTEIN, 30G CARBOHYDRATE, 7G TOTAL FAT (1G SATURATED), 4G FIBER, 0MG CHOLESTEROL, 257MG SODIUM.

TIP

Swap in 3 tablespoons Cilantro-Lime Dressing (page 35) for the oil, vinegar, salt, and pepper in step 4.

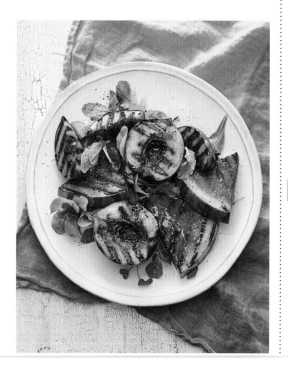

Fruit Meets Grill

Grilling fruit causes their natural sugars to caramelize, thereby deepening their flavor. That's welcome news if you're paleo and craving something sweet. Use this guide to grill-able fruits for your next salad—or dessert!

1 Prepare outdoor grill for direct grilling over medium heat.

2 Spray cut sides of fruit with nonstick cooking spray and place on hot grill rack.

3 Cook until grill marks appear, turning over once.

FRUIT	THICKNESS/SIZE	COOK	TIP
Apple	½-inch slices	4 to 6 minutes	Core fruit and slice into rings before grilling.
Apricot	Halved lengthwise	4 to 6 minutes	Toss with freshly grated lime zest after grilling.
Banana	Halved lengthwise	3 to 5 minutes	Remove skin after grilling, if you like.
Nectarine/ Peach/Plum	½-inch or 1-inch wedges	6 to 8 minutes	Remove skin after grilling, if you like.
Pineapple	½-inch slices or 1-inch wedges	5 to 10 minutes	Serve with lime wedges.
Strawberries	Whole	4 to 5 minutes	Thread on metal skewers.
Watermelon	½-inch wedges	3 to 4 minutes	Cool a few minutes before serving.

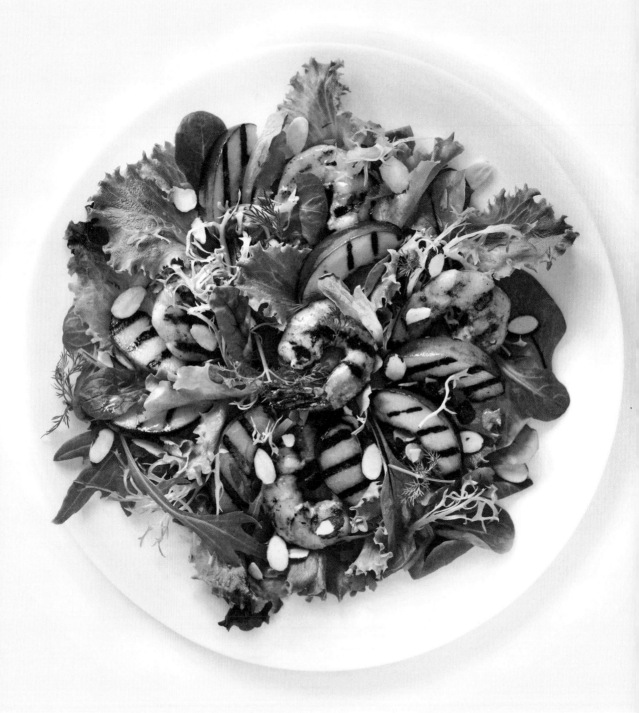

SHRIMP WITH
Grilled Nectarines

This hearty summer salad stars sweet grilled shrimp
and nectarines with creamy avocado and crunchy toasted nuts.
We toss the mix with a Classic Salad Dressing, but it's equally delish
with our Lemon-Oregano Dressing (page 35).

ACTIVE TIME: 20 MINUTES · **TOTAL TIME:** 30 MINUTES
MAKES: 4 MAIN-DISH SERVINGS

- 1 pound large shrimp, peeled and deveined
- 1 teaspoon olive or avocado oil
- ¼ teaspoon cayenne (ground red) pepper
- ⅛ teaspoon salt
- 2 nectarines, pitted and cut into thin wedges
- 6 ounces mixed salad greens
- ½ cup packed fresh basil leaves, thinly sliced
- ⅓ cup Classic Salad Dressing (page 35)
- 1 ripe avocado, sliced
- ¼ cup sliced almonds, toasted

1 Prepare outdoor grill for direct grilling over medium-high heat.

2 In large bowl, combine shrimp, oil, cayenne, and salt; toss to coat. Place shrimp on hot grill rack; cook for 3 to 5 minutes or until opaque throughout, turning over once. Transfer shrimp to plate and let cool for 5 minutes. Add nectarines to hot grill rack; cook for 4 minutes or until grill marks appear, turning over once.

3 In large bowl, combine greens, basil, and Classic Salad Dressing; toss to coat. Divide among four serving plates. Top evenly with shrimp, nectarines, avocado, and almonds.

EACH SERVING: ABOUT 400 CALORIES, 27G PROTEIN, 15G CARBOHYDRATE, 27G TOTAL FAT (4G SATURATED), 5G FIBER, 172MG CHOLESTEROL, 330MG SODIUM.

CHICKEN WITH
Grilled Nectarines

Prepare recipe as directed but substitute **1 pound boneless, skinless chicken breast halves** for shrimp. Prepare grill for covered direct grilling over medium heat. In large bowl, toss chicken, **2 teaspoons olive or avocado oil**; **1 teaspoon fresh thyme leaves**, chopped; **¼ teaspoon salt**; and **¼ teaspoon ground black pepper**. Place chicken on hot grill rack. Cover and cook for 11 to 13 minutes or until juices run clear when chicken is pierced with tip of knife, turning over once. Slice chicken.

EACH SERVING: ABOUT 415 CALORIES, 30G PROTEIN, 14G CARBOHYDRATE, 27G TOTAL FAT (4G SATURATED), 5G FIBER, 66MG CHOLESTEROL, 290MG SODIUM.

BALSAMIC ROASTED PORK
with Berry Salad

Quick-cooking pork tenderloin roasts with onion and fennel before being served atop a spinach-strawberry salad with balsamic vinaigrette and blackberries.

ACTIVE TIME: 25 MINUTES   **TOTAL TIME:** 35 MINUTES

MAKES: 4 MAIN-DISH SERVINGS

4 tablespoons balsamic vinegar

2 tablespoons extra-virgin olive oil

3 teaspoons Dijon mustard

2 teaspoons packed fresh oregano leaves, finely chopped

2 medium fennel bulbs, cut into ¼-inch-thick slices

1 small red onion (4 to 6 ounces), thinly sliced

1 whole pork tenderloin (1 pound), trimmed

Salt

⅛ teaspoon ground black pepper

1 pound strawberries

¼ cup packed fresh basil leaves

1 container (5 ounces) baby spinach

½ pint blackberries

1 Preheat oven to 450°F.

2 In large bowl with wire whisk, mix 3 tablespoons vinegar, 1 tablespoon oil, 2 teaspoons mustard, and oregano until well blended. Add fennel, tossing until well coated. Arrange on outer edges of 18" by 12" jelly-roll pan. To same bowl, add onions, tossing until well coated. Arrange onions in center of pan. Add pork to same bowl and toss until coated; place on top of onions.

3 Sprinkle pork and vegetables with ¼ teaspoon salt and pepper. Roast for 18 to 22 minutes or until meat thermometer inserted in thickest part of pork reaches 140°F. Let pork stand for 5 minutes to set juices for easier slicing.

4 While pork roasts, hull and slice strawberries. Finely chop basil; place in large bowl.

5 In bowl with basil, with wire whisk, mix remaining 1 tablespoon vinegar, 1 tablespoon oil, 1 teaspoon mustard, and ⅛ teaspoon salt until well blended. Thinly slice pork. Add fennel, onion, spinach, and strawberries to bowl with dressing; toss until well mixed. Divide among four serving plates. Top with blackberries and pork.

EACH SERVING: ABOUT 315 CALORIES, 26G PROTEIN, 30G CARBOHYDRATE, 11G TOTAL FAT (2G SATURATED), 10G FIBER, 62MG CHOLESTEROL, 480MG SODIUM.

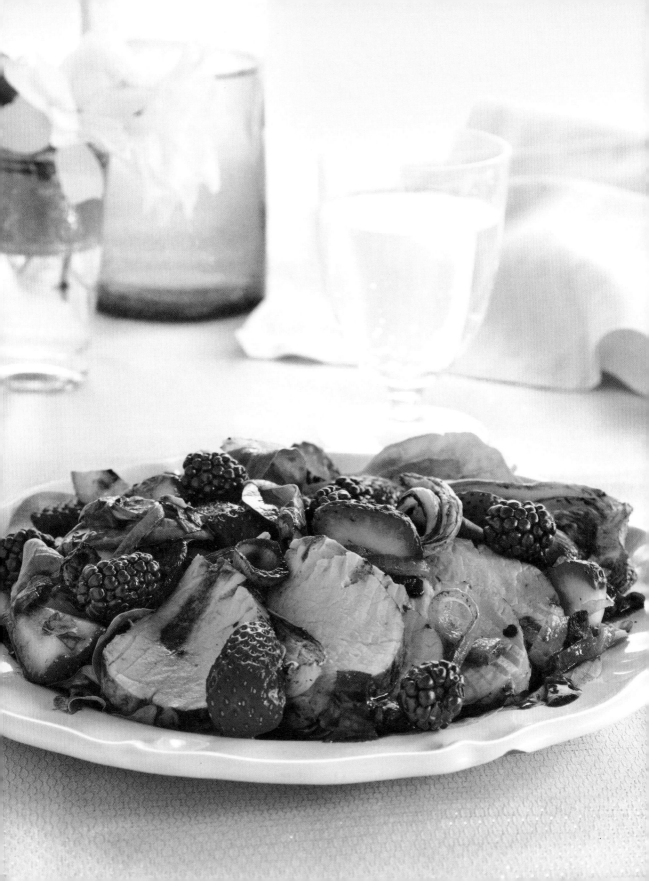

Summery Chicken
WALDORF SALAD

We turned the classic Waldorf salad into
a main dish by adding grilled chicken and veggies.
Light and refreshing, it's the perfect pick for an outdoor meal.

ACTIVE TIME: 20 MINUTES   **TOTAL TIME:** 45 MINUTES
MAKES: 4 MAIN-DISH SERVINGS

2 large yellow peppers, cut into quarters

1 pound boneless, skinless chicken breast
   halves

1 teaspoon olive or avocado oil

Salt

¼ teaspoon ground black pepper

¼ cup Rich Chicken Broth (page 14) or lower-
   sodium chicken broth

2 tablespoons fresh lemon juice

1 garlic clove, peeled

½ cup walnuts

2 medium stalks celery, finely chopped

½ cup seedless grapes, halved

1 container (10 ounces) mixed salad greens

1 Prepare outdoor grill for covered direct grilling
over medium-high heat.

2 Toss peppers and chicken with oil and ⅛
teaspoon salt. Place peppers and chicken on hot
grill rack; cook peppers, covered, for 10 minutes
or until charred, turning over once. Cover and
cook chicken for 12 to 15 minutes or until juices
run clear when chicken is pierced with tip of
knife, turning over once. Let cool.

3 In food processor with knife blade attached,
puree peppers, broth, lemon juice, garlic, ¼
teaspoon salt, and pepper. Add walnuts; pulse
until finely chopped.

4 Chop chicken; transfer to large bowl. Add
celery, grapes, and dressing; toss to coat. Serve
with greens.

EACH SERVING: ABOUT 271 CALORIES, 27G PROTEIN,
16G CARBOHYDRATE, 12G TOTAL FAT (2G SATURATED),
3G FIBER, 63MG CHOLESTEROL, 296MG SODIUM.

Tuscan Sun
SALMON SALAD

The salmon is steamed with sliced
lemon in the microwave, so it's a terrific
option for warm summer nights.

ACTIVE TIME: 10 MINUTES   **TOTAL TIME:** 15 MINUTES
MAKES: 4 MAIN-DISH SERVINGS

1   lemon, thinly sliced

4   pieces salmon fillet (5 ounces each), skin
    removed

¼   teaspoon salt

⅛   teaspoon ground black pepper

1   container (5 ounces) baby arugula

½   cup sliced roasted red peppers

½   cup pitted Kalamata olives

1   tablespoon balsamic vinegar

2   teaspoons extra-virgin olive, avocado,
    or flaxseed oil

1 In 8" by 8" glass baking dish, arrange lemon
slices in single layer. Add *¼ cup water.*

2 Place salmon fillets on top; sprinkle with salt
and pepper. Cover with vented plastic wrap and
microwave on high for 8 minutes or until fish is
just opaque throughout.

3 Meanwhile, in large bowl, toss arugula,
roasted peppers, olives, vinegar, and oil. Divide
among four serving plates and top with salmon.

EACH SERVING: ABOUT 257 CALORIES, 29G PROTEIN,
7G CARBOHYDRATE, 12G TOTAL FAT (2G SATURATED),
2G FIBER, 66MG CHOLESTEROL, 511MG SODIUM.

TIP

Ask for center-cut salmon fillets from your
fishmonger. Unlike thinner pieces from
the tail, these fillets will cook evenly in the
microwave.

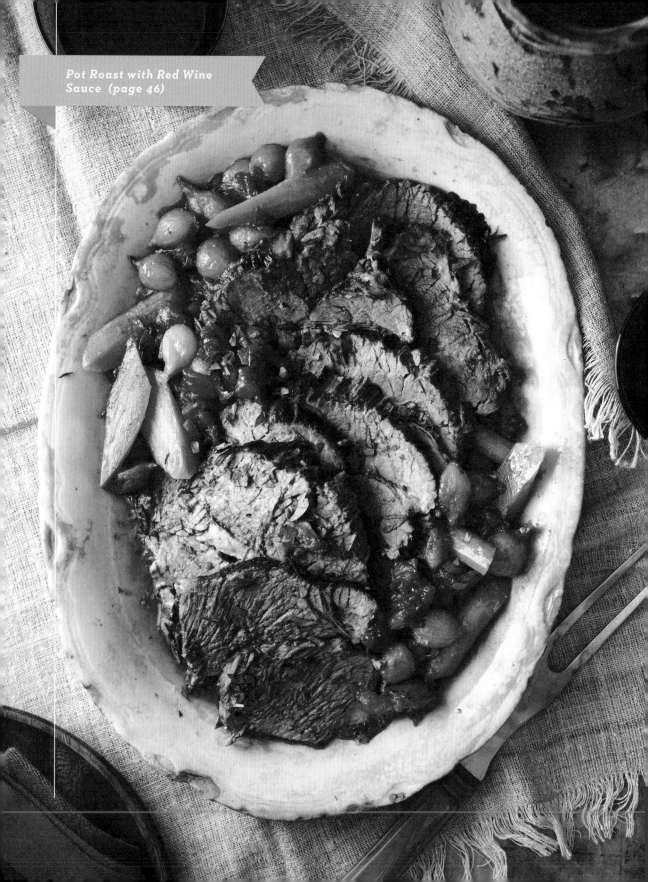

Pot Roast with Red Wine Sauce (page 46)

3 | Steaks, Chops & More

When you're eating paleo-style, lean protein takes center stage on the plate. And when it comes to smart meat choices, we've got an enticing collection to choose from. Love steak? Sink your teeth into our juicy Steak with Argentine Herb Sauce, Fire-Grilled Steak, or Pepper-Crusted Steak with Roasted Veggies. If you haven't tried pork tenderloin yet, our Pork & Gingered Apples and Curried Pork with Olives & Dried Plums will show you how easy and versatile this cut of meat can be. Plus, our Latin-Style Beef (Ropa Vieja), Pot Roast with Red Wine Sauce, and Lamb & Root Vegetable Tagine are custom-made for the slow cooker.

If your butcher has a selection of grass-fed beef, give it a try. Animals raised on grain and confined to feed lots have a higher fat content than grass-fed beef that's been pasture-raised. Grass-fed beef has a bolder, beefier flavor than conventional grain-fed beef, making it well worth the extra coin.

POT ROAST WITH
Red Wine Sauce

Prepare and serve this luscious dish
with an organic full-bodied red wine like
Cabernet or Pinot Noir. For photo, see page 44.

ACTIVE TIME: 20 MINUTES   **TOTAL TIME:** 10 HOURS 25 MINUTES
MAKES: 10 MAIN-DISH SERVINGS

1   boneless beef chuck roast (4½ pounds), tied

¾   teaspoon salt

¼   teaspoon ground black pepper

1   teaspoon olive oil

1   pound carrots

1   bag (16 ounces) frozen pearl onions

3   garlic cloves, crushed with press

½   teaspoon dried thyme

1   cup dry red wine

1   can (28 ounces) diced tomatoes, drained

1   bay leaf

Chopped fresh flat-leaf parsley leaves,
for garnish

1 With paper towels, pat beef dry; sprinkle all
over with salt and pepper.

2 In 12-inch skillet, heat oil over medium-high
heat until hot. Add beef and cook for 10 to 13
minutes, turning to brown all sides. Transfer to
6- to 6½-quart slow-cooker bowl.

3 While beef browns, peel carrots and cut into
2-inch chunks. Transfer to slow-cooker bowl.

4 To same skillet, add onions, garlic, and thyme.
Cook, stirring often, for 2 minutes or until
golden. Add wine; cook for 3 minutes, stirring
until browned bits are loosened from bottom of
pan. Transfer to slow-cooker bowl, along with
tomatoes and bay leaf. Cover slow-cooker and
cook on low for 10 hours.

5 Transfer beef to cutting board; discard strings.
Transfer vegetables to large serving platter;
discard bay leaf.

6 Transfer cooking liquid from slow-cooker bowl
to 8-cup liquid measuring cup; discard fat.

7 Slice meat across the grain and arrange on
serving platter with vegetables. Serve with
cooking liquid and garnish with parsley.

EACH SERVING: ABOUT 515 CALORIES, 47G PROTEIN,
11G CARBOHYDRATE, 30G TOTAL FAT (12G SATURATED),
3G FIBER, 181MG CHOLESTEROL, 205MG SODIUM.

TIP
This dish can be refrigerated in an airtight
container for up to 3 days.

LATIN-STYLE BEEF
(Ropa Vieja)

Ropa Vieja is a classic Cuban beef stew with a spicy tomato sauce. Simmered for hours, the beef is then shredded so it resembles "old clothes," hence the name. Our version is slow-cooker simple.

ACTIVE TIME: 20 MINUTES   **TOTAL TIME:** 9 HOURS 20 MINUTES
MAKES: 8 MAIN-DISH SERVINGS

- 1 can (14½ ounces) diced tomatoes
- 1 tablespoon capers, drained
- 1 tablespoon ground cumin
- 1 teaspoon salt
- ½ teaspoon ground cinnamon
- 3 garlic cloves, sliced
- 2 large red, yellow, and/or green peppers, sliced
- 2 large pickled jalapeño chiles, sliced
- 1 medium onion, sliced
- 1 fresh beef brisket (about 3 pounds)

1 In 4½- to 6-quart slow-cooker bowl, combine tomatoes with their juices, capers, cumin, salt, and cinnamon. Add garlic, peppers, jalapeños, onion, and brisket; stir to coat brisket and vegetables with tomato mixture. Cover slow-cooker and cook on low for 9 to 10 hours or on high for 6 to 6½ hours.

2 With slotted spoon, transfer brisket and vegetables to large bowl. With two forks, shred brisket with the grain into fine strips. Skim and discard fat from cooking liquid. Stir cooking liquid into brisket mixture.

EACH SERVING: ABOUT 400 CALORIES, 35G PROTEIN, 7G CARBOHYDRATE, 25G TOTAL FAT (9G SATURATED), 2G FIBER, 109MG CHOLESTEROL, 690MG SODIUM.

TIP

To prep this dish ahead, premeasure the ingredients, precut the vegetables, trim the brisket, and mix the liquids and seasonings. Refrigerate the components separately in bowls or self-sealing plastic bags overnight.

Fire-Grilled
STEAK

Juicy flank steak is paired with grilled sweet fennel and onion,
then topped with a refreshing mint vinaigrette.

ACTIVE TIME: 15 MINUTES   **TOTAL TIME:** 35 MINUTES
MAKES: 4 MAIN-DISH SERVINGS

1   beef flank steak (1 pound)

Salt

¼   teaspoon ground black pepper

5   teaspoons extra-virgin olive oil

2   medium fennel bulbs, cored and cut
     lengthwise into ½-inch-thick slices

1   large red onion (8 to 10 ounces), cut into
     ⅓-inch-thick rounds

½   cup fresh mint leaves

½   cup fresh flat-leaf parsley leaves

3   tablespoons red wine vinegar

2   tablespoons capers, rinsed and drained

1   small garlic clove, crushed with press

1 Prepare outdoor grill for covered direct grilling
over medium heat. Sprinkle steak with ¼ teaspoon
salt and pepper. Use 2 teaspoons oil to brush both
sides of fennel and onion slices; sprinkle with
⅛ teaspoon salt.

2 Place onion and steaks on hot grill rack. Cook
onion, covered, for 7 to 9 minutes or until tender,
turning over once. Cover and cook steak for 8
to 10 minutes for medium-rare or until desired
doneness, turning over once. Transfer onion to
bowl. Transfer steak to cutting board; let stand
for 10 minutes to set juices for easier slicing.

3 Meanwhile, finely chop mint and parsley;
place in medium bowl with vinegar, capers,

1 tablespoon water, garlic, and remaining
3 teaspoons oil. Stir to blend.

4 Place fennel on hot grill rack. Cover and cook
for 3 to 4 minutes or until browned, turning over
once. Toss with onion.

5 Thinly slice steak across the grain. Serve with
fennel, onion, and vinaigrette.

....

EACH SERVING: ABOUT 290 CALORIES, 26G PROTEIN,
16G CARBOHYDRATE, 13G TOTAL FAT (4G SATURATED),
6G FIBER, 67MG CHOLESTEROL, 465MG SODIUM.

The Tender Cut

You've heard it before: When ready to carve
a piece of meat, the recipe says, "Slice across
the grain." But what does that mean and why
is it important? For recipes like our Fire-
Grilled Steak or Pot Roast with Red Wine
Sauce (page 46), look closely and you'll notice
long lines at the top of the meat. Those are
fibers of muscle running through the meat.
If you slice in the same direction as the lines,
you'll have to chew through the tough fibers.
But if you thinly slice across the grain, the
carving (versus your chewing) will produce
smaller fibers, so you can enjoy tender slices
of beef on your plate.

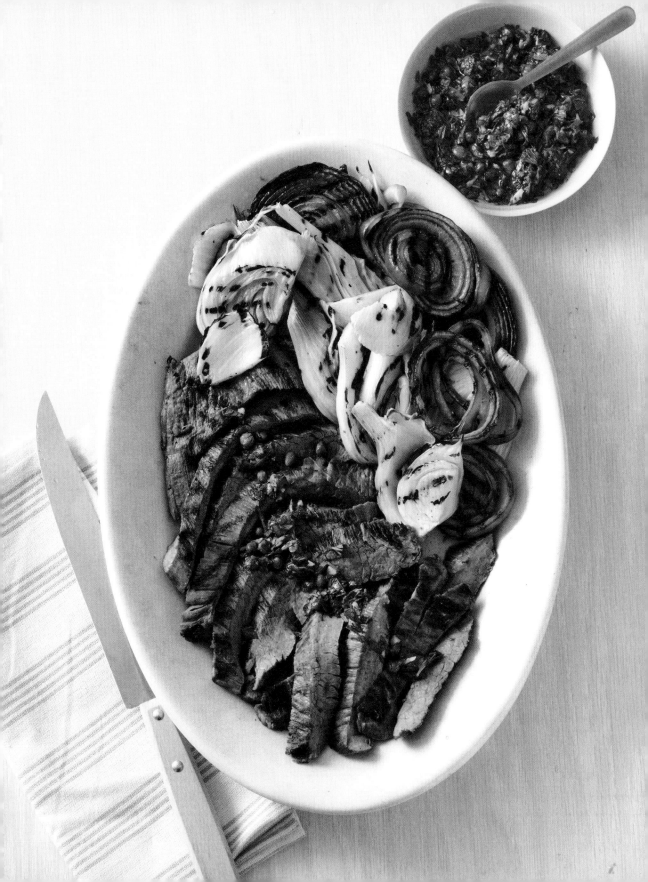

SPICED MEATBALLS
with Saucy Tomatoes

Serve these tender meatballs seasoned with parsley, cumin, and oregano with a side of spaghetti squash.

ACTIVE TIME: 15 MINUTES   **TOTAL TIME:** 35 MINUTES
MAKES: 4 MAIN-DISH SERVINGS

1   pound ground beef chuck

2   garlic cloves, crushed with press

3   tablespoons packed fresh flat-leaf parsley leaves, finely chopped, plus additional for garnish

1   teaspoon ground cumin

1   cup finely chopped onion

1½ teaspoons dried oregano

½   teaspoon salt

½   teaspoon ground black pepper

1   tablespoon olive oil

2   pints grape tomatoes

2   ounces feta cheese, crumbled (½ cup)

1   In large bowl, with hands, combine beef, garlic, parsley, cumin, ½ cup onion, 1 teaspoon oregano, salt, and pepper until well mixed.

2   With wet hands, shape mixture into 12 small (2-inch round, 1-inch high), slightly flattened meatballs.

3   In 12-inch skillet, heat oil over medium-high heat until hot. Add meatballs in single layer. Cook for 8 to 9 minutes, or until browned and instant-read thermometer inserted in center reaches 160°F, turning over once. Transfer meatballs to plate.

4   Drain fat from skillet and discard. To same skillet, add remaining ½ cup onion; cook, stirring, over medium-high heat for 1 minute. Add tomatoes and remaining ½ teaspoon oregano. Cook, stirring occasionally, for 5 to 7 minutes or until tomatoes soften and some burst.

5   To serve, divide meatballs and tomato mixture among serving plates. Sprinkle with feta and garnish with parsley.

EACH SERVING: ABOUT 320 CALORIES, 24G PROTEIN, 11G CARBOHYDRATE, 20G TOTAL FAT (8G SATURATED), 3G FIBER, 79MG CHOLESTEROL, 456MG SODIUM.

TIP

These meatballs can be covered and refrigerated overnight before cooking. If making ahead, increase the cooking time by 5 minutes in step 3.

STEAK WITH
Argentine Herb Sauce

Chimichurri is a green sauce from Argentina that's served with grilled meat. Our version is a combo of fresh parsley and cilantro spiked with sherry vinegar and crushed red pepper.

ACTIVE TIME: 15 MINUTES   **TOTAL TIME:** 25 MINUTES
MAKES: 6 MAIN-DISH SERVINGS

1   cup packed fresh flat-leaf parsley leaves

1   cup packed fresh cilantro leaves

1   garlic clove

3   tablespoons extra-virgin olive oil

2   tablespoons sherry vinegar

¼   teaspoon dried oregano

¼   teaspoon crushed red pepper

Kosher salt and ground black pepper

4   New York beef strip steaks (2½ pounds total), each 1-inch thick

1   Prepare outdoor grill for direct grilling over medium-high heat. Fit wire rack into jelly-roll pan.

2   Prepare herb sauce: In food processor with knife blade attached, combine parsley, cilantro, and garlic; pulse until finely chopped. Add oil, vinegar, oregano, crushed red pepper, and ⅛ teaspoon each salt and pepper; pulse to blend.

3   Pat steaks dry. Sprinkle steaks with ½ teaspoon each salt and pepper. Immediately place steaks on hot grill rack. Cook for 7 to 8 minutes for medium-rare or until desired doneness, turning over every 2 to 3 minutes. Transfer to wire rack. Let stand for 5 minutes to set juices for easier slicing.

4   Stir any meat juices into herb sauce. Slice steak across grain; serve with sauce.

EACH SERVING: ABOUT 445 CALORIES, 38G PROTEIN, 1G CARBOHYDRATE, 31G TOTAL FAT (10G SATURATED), 1G FIBER, 136MG CHOLESTEROL, 285MG SODIUM.

Rosemary-Lemon
STEAK

Prepare recipe as directed but omit herb sauce and salt and pepper for steaks. In bowl, combine **1 tablespoon minced fresh rosemary, 1½ teaspoons freshly grated lemon peel, 2 teaspoons kosher salt**, and **½ teaspoon ground black pepper**. Cut **1 garlic clove** in half; rub cut sides all over steaks. Sprinkle rosemary mixture all over steaks; pat into meat. Grill as directed.

EACH SERVING: ABOUT 375 CALORIES, 38G PROTEIN, 0G CARBOHYDRATE, 24G TOTAL FAT (9G SATURATED), 0G FIBER, 136MG CHOLESTEROL, 720MG SODIUM.

TIP

New York beef strip steaks can be sold by several names: club steak, Kansas City steak, or top loin steak.

STEAK WITH
Broccolini-Radish Salad

Filet mignon steaks, roasted sweet potato, and broccoli
are all topped with an elegant red wine and thyme pan sauce.

ACTIVE TIME: 10 MINUTES **TOTAL TIME:** 25 MINUTES
MAKES: 4 MAIN-DISH SERVINGS

2 boneless beef sirloin steaks, 1³/₄ pounds
   (each about 1¹/₂ inches thick)

1 teaspoon salt

¹/₂ teaspoon ground black pepper

2 bunches broccolini, trimmed

2 tablespoons olive oil

2 tablespoons Dijon mustard

2 tablespoons lemon juice

5 radishes, sliced

2 green onions, thinly sliced

1 Prepare outdoor grill for covered direct
grilling over medium-high heat.

2 Sprinkle steaks with ¹/₂ teaspoon salt and
pepper. Place steaks on hot grill rack. Cook for
10 minutes for medium-rare or until desired
doneness, turning over once. Transfer steaks to
cutting board. Let stand 10 minutes to set juices
for easier slicing.

3 In large bowl, toss broccolini, 1 tablespoon
oil, and ¹/₄ teaspoon salt. Place broccolini on hot
grill rack; cover and cook, turning occasionally,
for 4 minutes or until tender.

4 Meanwhile, make dressing: In large bowl
with wire whisk, mix mustard, lemon juice,
and remaining 1 tablespoon olive oil and
¹/₄ teaspoon salt.

5 Slice steak across grain. Add broccolini,
radishes, and green onions to dressing; toss
to coat and serve with steak.

EACH SERVING: ABOUT 476 CALORIES, 40G PROTEIN,
13G CARBOHYDRATE, 29G TOTAL FAT (9G SATURATED),
5G FIBER, 118MG CHOLESTEROL, 841MG SODIUM.

TIP

Broccolini, a cross between broccoli and
Chinese broccoli, is milder than regular
broccoli with a sweet, earthy taste. Its
slender stalks are also completely edible.

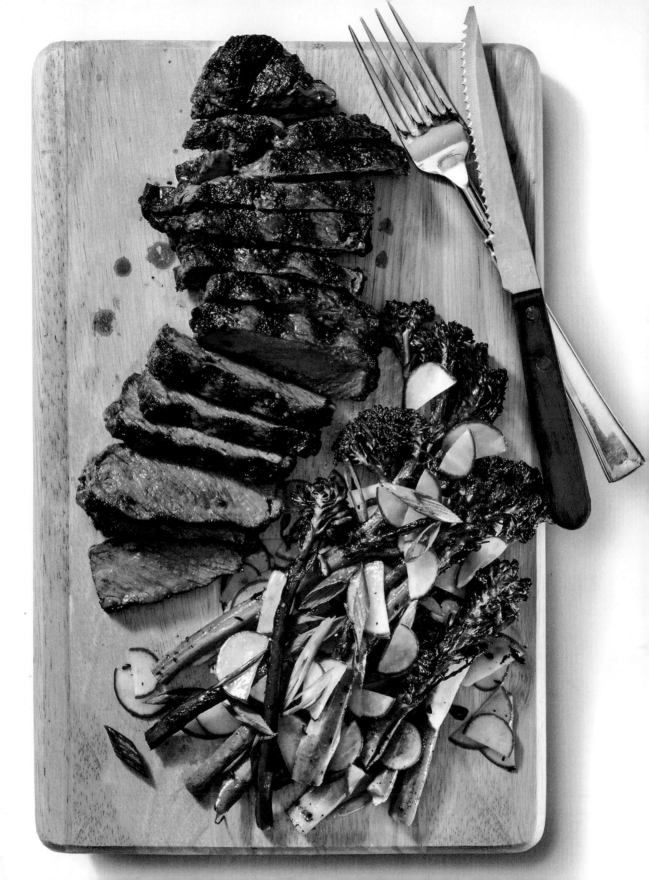

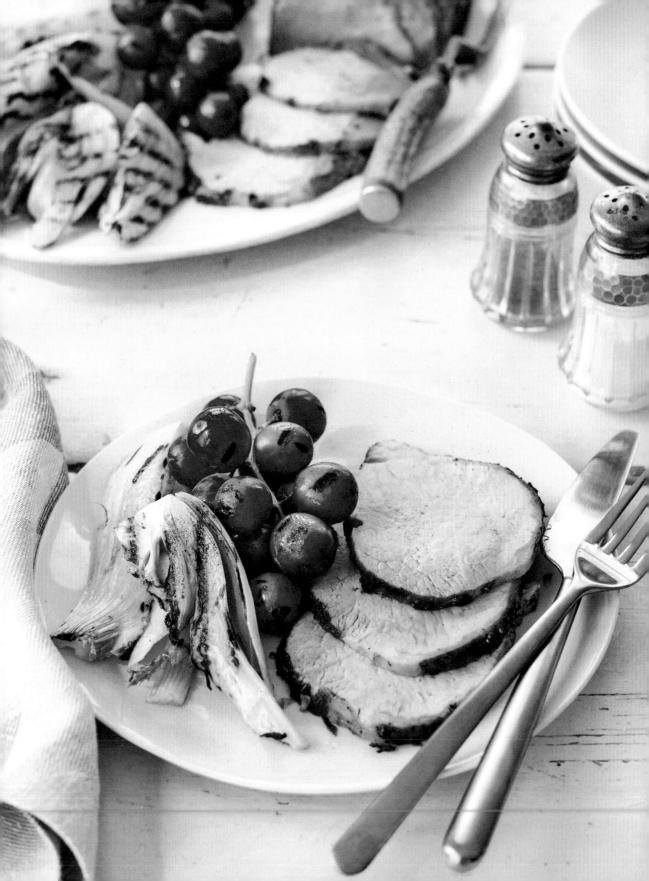

PORK LOIN WITH
Lemon, Thyme & Garlic

The aroma of this fragrant grilled roast is sure to
bring everyone to the table.

ACTIVE TIME: 15 MINUTES   **TOTAL TIME:** 1 HOUR PLUS STANDING
MAKES: 8 MAIN-DISH SERVINGS

4   lemons

4   garlic cloves, crushed with press

2   tablespoons fresh thyme leaves, chopped

1   tablespoon olive oil

1/2   teaspoon salt

1/2   teaspoon coarsely ground black pepper

1   boneless pork loin roast (3 pounds)

1 Prepare outdoor grill for covered indirect grilling over medium heat.

2 From 2 lemons, grate 1 tablespoon peel and squeeze 1 tablespoon juice. Cut each remaining lemon into 4 wedges.

3 In small bowl, combine lemon peel and juice, garlic, thyme, oil, salt, and pepper.

4 Make 10 to 12 (1-inch-long and 1/2-inch-deep) slits in pork. Rub pork all over with lemon mixture, pushing some into slits.

5 Place pork on hot grill rack. Cook over direct heat for 10 minutes, turning several times to sear all sides. Move pork to unheated burner; cover and cook for about 35 minutes or until meat thermometer inserted into center of pork reaches 140°F. Transfer pork to cutting board; let stand for 10 minutes to set juices for easier slicing. (Internal temperature of pork will rise 5 to 10 degrees upon standing.)

6 Serve sliced pork with lemon wedges and any juices from cutting board.

EACH SERVING: ABOUT 350 CALORIES, 35G PROTEIN, 3G CARBOHYDRATE, 21G TOTAL FAT (7G SATURATED), 1G FIBER, 112MG CHOLESTEROL, 240MG SODIUM.

TIP

Pair this roast with Smoky Paprika Grapes (page 112) for a magnificent company meal.

PORK &
Gingered Apples

Gently spiced with coriander and cumin,
sautéed pork is topped with a compote
of sweet apples and grated fresh ginger.

ACTIVE TIME: 10 MINUTES   **TOTAL TIME:** 30 MINUTES
MAKES: 4 MAIN-DISH SERVINGS

½ teaspoon ground coriander

¼ teaspoon ground cumin

Salt

¼ teaspoon ground black pepper

1 whole pork tenderloin (1 pound), trimmed

2 teaspoons olive oil

3 Gala or Fuji apples, cored

2 garlic cloves, crushed with press

1 teaspoon grated, peeled fresh ginger

1 In small bowl, combine ¼ teaspoon coriander, ⅛ teaspoon cumin, ⅛ teaspoon salt, and pepper. Cut pork tenderloin crosswise into 1½-inch-thick slices. Press each slice with hand to flatten slightly; rub with spices.

2 In 12-inch skillet, heat oil over medium-high heat until hot. Add pork; cook for 4 minutes or until golden. Turn pork; cook for 3 to 4 minutes more or until barely pink in center. Transfer to plate.

3 Meanwhile, coarsely grate one apple and chop remaining two apples.

4 Reduce heat to medium. Add garlic and ginger; cook, stirring often, until fragrant, about 30 seconds. Add apples and remaining ¼ teaspoon coriander and ⅛ teaspoon cumin. Cook, stirring often, for 2 minutes. Add *1 cup water* and ¼ teaspoon salt, stirring until browned bits are loosened from bottom of pan. Cover and cook for 7 minutes or until apples are very tender. Return pork to skillet; cook for 2 minutes more or until heated through.

EACH SERVING: ABOUT 310 CALORIES, 28G PROTEIN, 40G CARBOHYDRATE, 5G TOTAL FAT (1G SATURATED), 8G FIBER, 74MG CHOLESTEROL, 285MG SODIUM.

 TIP
This dish pairs perfectly with wilted Swiss chard, baby kale, or spinach.

CURRIED PORK WITH
Olives & Dried Plums

Curry is often paired with fruit, and for this simple
dish we chose lusciously rich dried plums.
Stuffed olives give the sauce an unexpected flavor boost.

ACTIVE TIME: 5 MINUTES   **TOTAL TIME:** 25 MINUTES
MAKES: 6 MAIN-DISH SERVINGS

2   whole pork tenderloins (¾ pound each)

1   tablespoon curry powder

1   teaspoon coconut or olive oil

1¾ cups Rich Chicken Broth (page 14) or 1 can
     (14½ ounces) lower-sodium chicken broth

½   cup pitted dried plums (prunes)

¼   cup chopped pimiento-stuffed olives

1 Rub pork with curry powder. In 10-inch
nonstick skillet, heat oil over medium-high heat
until hot. Add pork and cook for 5 to 7 minutes,
turning to brown all sides. Add broth, dried plums,
and olives; heat to boiling. Partially cover skillet
and cook for about 10 minutes, turning pork
occasionally, or until meat thermometer inserted
into center of pork reaches 140°F.

2 Transfer pork to cutting board; let stand
for 5 minutes to set juices for easier slicing.
Meanwhile, add dried plums and olives to pan
juices; cover and keep warm.

3 Slice pork and serve with dried plums, olives,
and pan juices.

EACH SERVING: ABOUT 187 CALORIES, 24G PROTEIN,
10G CARBOHYDRATE, 6G TOTAL FAT (2G SATURATED),
2G FIBER, 74MG CHOLESTEROL, 301MG SODIUM.

TIP
Sprinkle each serving with chopped fresh
cilantro, if desired.

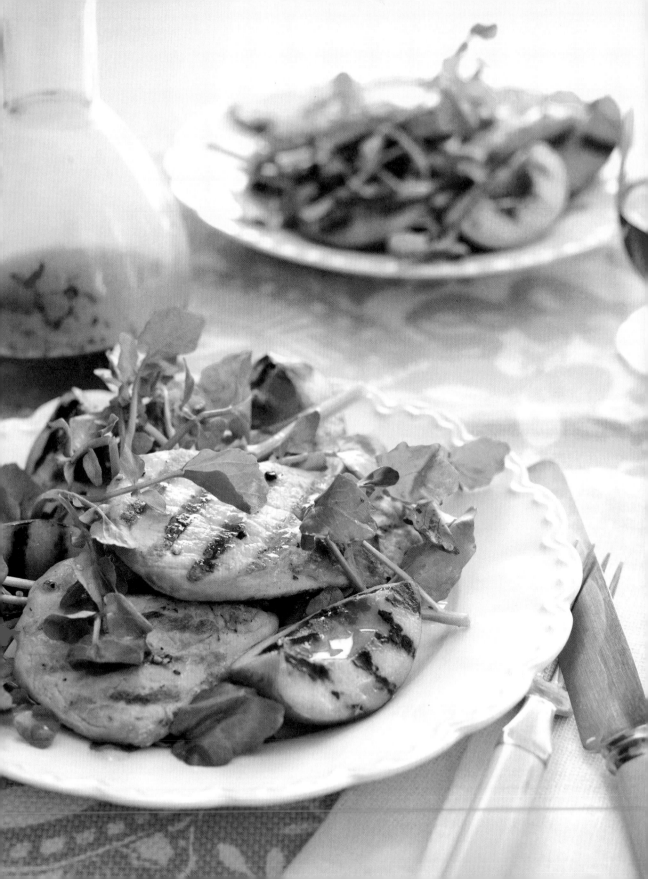

PORK TENDERLOIN
with Nectarines

This pork dinner is custom-made for a ridged grill pan. It's also terrific with grilled peaches.

ACTIVE TIME: 15 MINUTES   **TOTAL TIME:** 35 MINUTES
MAKES: 4 MAIN-DISH SERVINGS

4   ripe but firm nectarines, pitted and cut into 4 wedges

1   teaspoon plus 2 tablespoons olive oil

½   teaspoon salt

Ground black pepper

1   whole pork tenderloin (1¼ pounds), trimmed

2   tablespoons white balsamic vinegar

1   bunch watercress (6 ounces), rinsed with tough stems trimmed and discarded

1   Heat large ridged grill pan over medium heat until hot. Brush nectarine wedges with 1 teaspoon oil and sprinkle with ⅛ teaspoon each salt and pepper. Place nectarine wedges in grill pan and cook for about 10 minutes or until charred and tender, turning wedges over once. Transfer nectarines to plate and cover with foil to keep warm.

2   Meanwhile, cut pork tenderloin crosswise into 8 equal pieces. With palm of hand, firmly press on cut side of each piece to flatten to about a 1-inch-thick medallion. Sprinkle pork with ¼ teaspoon salt and ⅛ teaspoon pepper.

3   To same grill pan, add pork and cook for about 10 to 12 minutes or until browned on the outside and still slightly pink in the center, turning over once.

4   While pork is cooking, make dressing: In small bowl with wire whisk, mix vinegar, remaining ⅛ teaspoon salt, ⅛ teaspoon pepper, and remaining 2 tablespoons oil until well blended. Makes ¼ cup. Remove 1 tablespoon dressing; set aside.

5   In large bowl, toss watercress and remaining dressing. Place on four serving plates and top with pork and nectarines. Drizzle pork with reserved dressing.

....

EACH SERVING: ABOUT 325 CALORIES, 32G PROTEIN, 18G CARBOHYDRATE, 14G TOTAL FAT (3G SATURATED), 3G FIBER, 89MG CHOLESTEROL, 380MG SODIUM.

PORK MEDALLIONS
with Melon Salsa & Grilled Limes

Lime, melons, and a jalapeño chile bring Caribbean sizzle to a pork dinner—along with loads of vitamins A and C.

TOTAL TIME: 30 MINUTES **MAKES:** 4 MAIN-DISH SERVINGS

1 whole pork tenderloin, trimmed of fat (1¼ pounds total)

4 to 5 limes

1 tablespoon olive oil

½ cup loosely packed fresh cilantro leaves, chopped

¼ teaspoon salt

⅛ teaspoon coarsely ground black pepper

2 cups cantaloupe, chopped

1 cup honeydew melon, chopped

1 jalapeño chile, minced

1 Prepare outdoor grill for direct grilling over medium heat.

2 Cut pork tenderloin crosswise into 8 equal pieces. With palm of hand, firmly press on cut side of each piece to flatten into about 1-inch-thick medallion.

3 Cut 2 limes in half; reserve for grilling. From remaining limes, grate 1 teaspoon peel and squeeze ¼ cup juice. In small bowl, combine oil, ½ teaspoon lime peel, ¼ cup cilantro, ⅛ teaspoon salt, and pepper. Rub mixture on pork medallions to season both sides.

4 Place pork on hot grill; cook for 4 minutes. Turn pork over. Add lime halves, cut-sides down, to same grill grate; cook for 3 to 4 minutes or until lightly browned and warm. Cook pork for 4 to 5 minutes longer or until browned on the outside and still slightly pink in the center.

5 Meanwhile, in medium bowl, combine melons, jalapeño, lime juice, and remaining salt, cilantro, and lime peel. Makes about 3 cups salsa.

6 Serve pork with melon salsa and grilled limes (to squeeze over pork).

EACH SERVING: ABOUT 240 CALORIES, 31G PROTEIN, 17G CARBOHYDRATE, 8G TOTAL FAT (2G SATURATED), 2G FIBER, 78MG CHOLESTEROL, 225MG SODIUM.

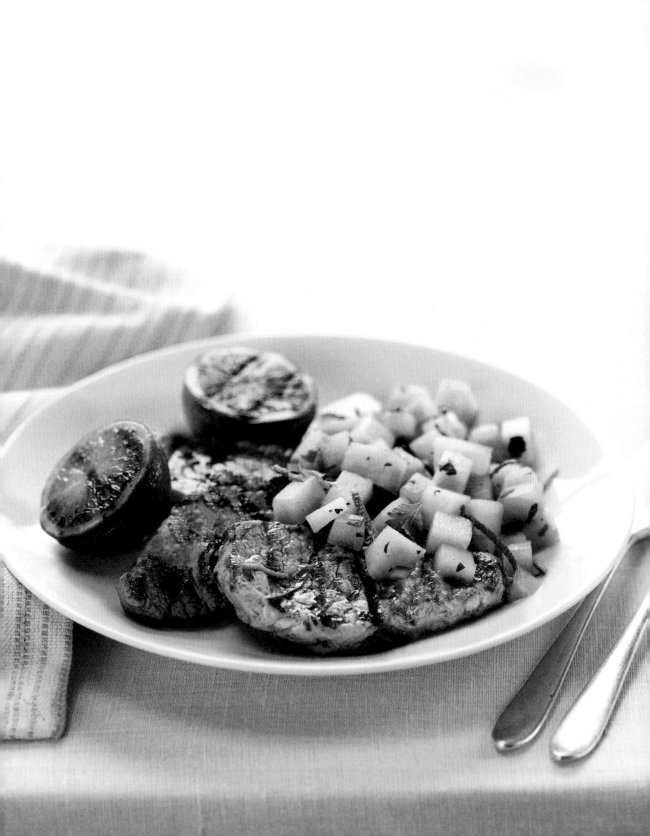

LAMB & ROOT VEGETABLE
Tagine

Tagine, a traditional stew from North Africa, is known for its combination of sweet and salty ingredients. This slow-cooker version includes dried apricots, lamb shoulder, and heaps of root vegetables.

ACTIVE TIME: 30 MINUTES **TOTAL TIME:** 8 HOURS 30 MINUTES
MAKES: 10 MAIN-DISH SERVINGS

1 tablespoon olive oil

4 pounds well-trimmed boneless lamb leg, cut into 1-inch chunks

½ teaspoon salt

¼ teaspoon ground black pepper

1¾ cups Rich Chicken Broth (page 14) or 1 can (14½ ounces) lower-sodium chicken broth

1 medium onion, chopped

2 garlic cloves, thinly sliced

1 pound sweet potatoes (2 medium), peeled and cut into 1-inch chunks

1 pound parsnips (6 medium), peeled and cut into 1-inch chunks

½ cup dried apricots, cut in half

2 teaspoons ground coriander

2 teaspoons ground cumin

¼ teaspoon ground cinnamon

½ cup pitted green olives, coarsely chopped

Fresh cilantro leaves, for garnish

1 In 12-inch skillet, heat oil over medium-high heat until very hot. Sprinkle lamb with salt and pepper. Add lamb to skillet in 3 batches, and cook for 5 to 6 minutes per batch or until lamb is browned on all sides, stirring occasionally and adding more oil if necessary. With slotted spoon, transfer lamb to medium bowl once browned.

2 After all lamb is browned, add broth to same skillet and heat to boiling over high heat, stirring until browned bits are loosened from bottom of pan. Boil for 1 minute.

3 Meanwhile, in 6- to 6½-quart slow-cooker bowl, combine onion, garlic, sweet potatoes, parsnips, apricots, coriander, cumin, and cinnamon. Top with browned lamb, any juices in bowl, and broth mixture; do not stir. Cover slow cooker and cook on low for 8 hours.

4 Skim and discard fat from cooking liquid. Stir olives into lamb mixture in slow cooker. Divide tagine among serving bowls. Garnish with cilantro leaves.

....

EACH SERVING: ABOUT 332 CALORIES, 31G PROTEIN, 20G CARBOHYDRATE, 14G TOTAL FAT (4G SATURATED), 4G FIBER, 99MG CHOLESTEROL, 342MG SODIUM.

TIP

If the lamb is not well trimmed when you buy it, purchase 5 pounds and cut away the excess fat yourself in order to yield 4 pounds of solid meat.

Slow Good

Before you make our slow-cooker Latin-Style Beef (page 47),
Pot Roast with Red Wine Sauce (page 46), or Lamb & Root Vegetable
Tagine (at left), follow these steps to succeed:

PREP SMART. Fat retains heat better than water. That means foods high in fat, like meat, will cook in a slow cooker faster than less fatty foods, like vegetables. To make sure your ingredients are evenly cooked, cut any vegetables—particularly root vegetables—into pieces that are a bit smaller than those you cut the meat into.

FILL 'ER UP. Fill the slow cooker at least half full but no more than three-quarters full (just be sure to leave 2 inches between the food and the lid). Put the ingredients that take the longest to cook—like root vegetables—on the bottom and along the sides of the bowl for maximum heat exposure. Place quicker-cooking ingredients toward the center.

KEEP A LID ON IT. Each time you uncover the slow cooker and stir its contents, the internal temperature drops by 10° to 15°F (thus requiring the cooking time to increase by 20 to 30 minutes). If you wish to check for doneness toward the end of the cooking time, replace the lid as quickly as possible.

TOO MUCH COOKING LIQUID? Remove the solids to a serving dish with a slotted spoon and keep warm. Turn the slow cooker on high; cook the remaining liquid, uncovered, to reduce to the desired thickness.

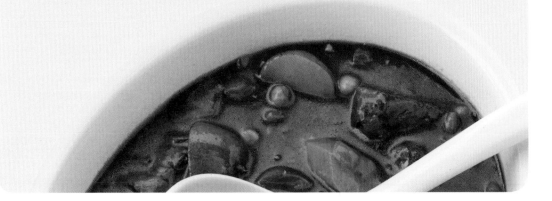

BUTTERFLIED LEG OF LAMB
with Mint Pesto

Juicy, chargrilled leg of lamb is topped with a
fresh mint-and-almond pesto for a flavor match made in heaven.
Complete the meal with Vegetable Kebabs (page 122).

ACTIVE TIME: 20 MINUTES **TOTAL TIME:** 45 MINUTES PLUS CHILLING
MAKES: 12 MAIN-DISH SERVINGS

4½ cups loosely packed fresh mint leaves

2   garlic cloves, crushed with press

⅓   cup olive oil

1   teaspoon salt

1   teaspoon coarsely ground black pepper

4   pounds boneless butterflied leg of lamb,
     trimmed

¾   cup almonds

1 In food processor with knife blade attached,
pulse mint leaves, garlic, ½ *cup water*, oil, salt,
and pepper until well blended.
2 Place lamb in 13" by 9" glass baking dish.
Remove ¼ cup mint mixture from food processor;
spread on lamb to coat both sides. Cover and
refrigerate for at least 1 hour or up to 6 hours.
3 Meanwhile, add almonds to mint mixture
remaining in food processor and pulse until almonds
are finely chopped. Spoon pesto into serving bowl;
cover and refrigerate until ready to serve.

4 Remove lamb from refrigerator about 15
minutes before cooking. Prepare outdoor grill for
direct covered grilling over medium heat.
5 Place lamb on hot grill rack. Cover and cook
for 20 to 35 minutes (depending on thickness) for
medium-rare, turning lamb over once halfway
through cooking and removing pieces to cutting
board as they are done. When remaining lamb
is done, transfer to same cutting board and
let stand for 10 minutes to set juices for easier
slicing. Serve lamb with mint pesto and any juices
from cutting board.

EACH SERVING: ABOUT 380 CALORIES, 32G PROTEIN,
5G CARBOHYDRATE, 26G TOTAL FAT (8G SATURATED),
4G FIBER, 99MG CHOLESTEROL, 270MG SODIUM.

TIP

The thickness of a butterflied leg of lamb
will vary; check thinner pieces early for
doneness, cut off those sections as they are
cooked, and place them on a cutting board.
Cover with foil to keep warm.

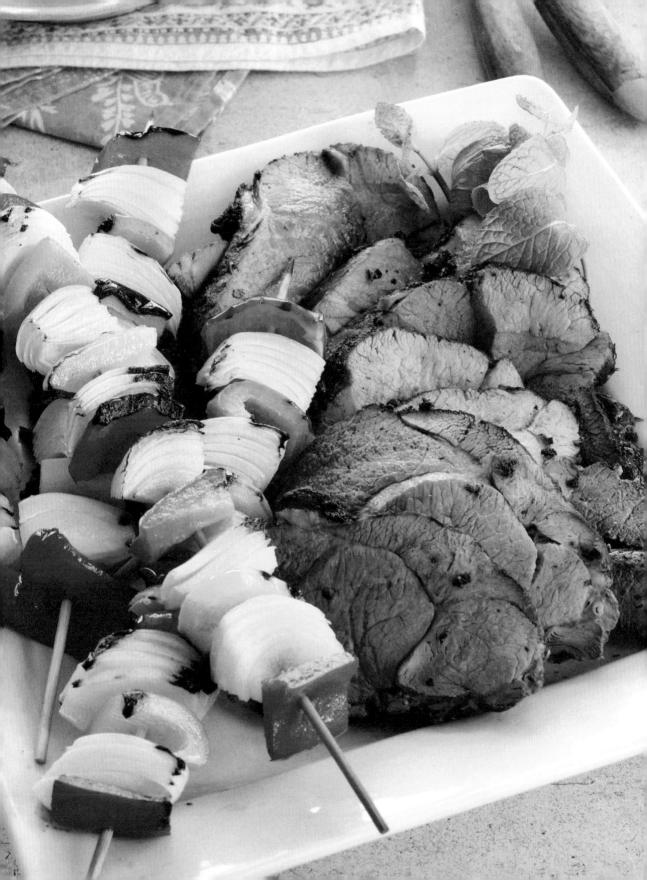

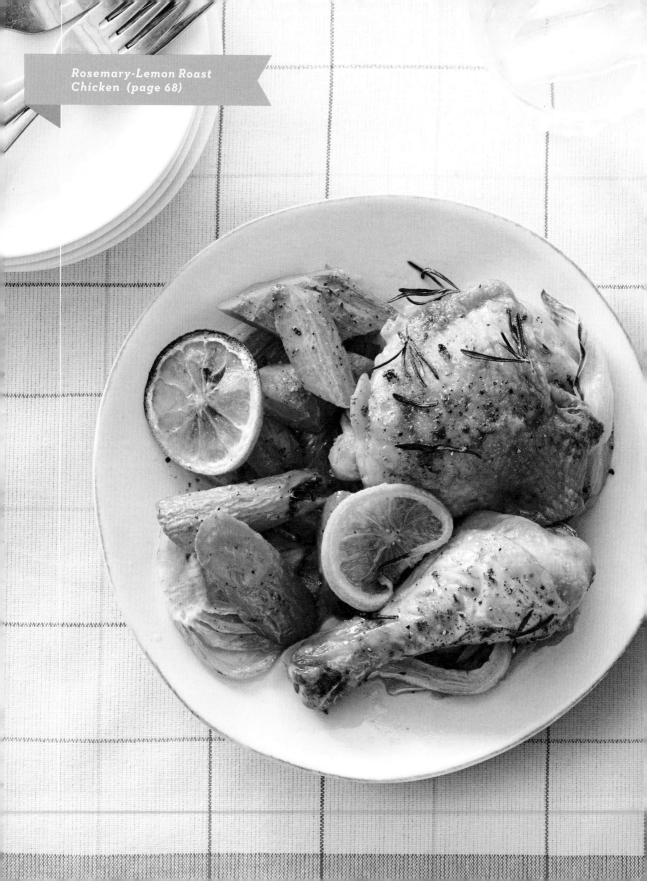

Rosemary-Lemon Roast
Chicken (page 68)

4 Best-Ever Chicken

Chicken *again*? No problem—especially if you're following the paleo plan. Our selection of fabulous chicken (and turkey) dishes offers lots of great ideas. We're serving up flash-in-the-pan dishes like Grilled Chicken & Greens, Chicken with Orange Relish, or Tarragon Turkey with Grapes—all ready in 30 minutes (or less)—along with Chicken with Caramelized Cauliflower & Green Olives, Caribbean Chicken Thighs, or Coconut-Curry Chicken for more adventurous diners. Best of all, thanks to our trio of salt-free rubs, it only takes a sprinkle and a bird to get dinner on the table any night of the week.

Rosemary-Lemon
ROAST CHICKEN

Drumsticks and thighs roasted with lemon and herbs sit atop
a bed of carrots and fennel. For photo, see page 66.

ACTIVE TIME: 15 MINUTES   **TOTAL TIME:** 45 MINUTES
MAKES: 4 MAIN-DISH SERVINGS

1   pound carrots, cut into 2-inch lengths

1   pound fennel, trimmed and thinly sliced

2   tablespoons olive oil

¾   teaspoon salt

8   small chicken pieces (drumsticks and thighs),
    patted dry (about 3 pounds total)

2   lemons

2   tablespoons loosely packed rosemary leaves

½   teaspoon ground black pepper

1   Preheat oven to 475°F.

2   In large roasting pan or rimmed baking sheet,
toss carrots, fennel, oil, and ¼ teaspoon salt;
spread in single layer. Arrange chicken on top
of vegetables.

3   From lemons, grate peel all over chicken.
Sprinkle chicken with rosemary, remaining
½ teaspoon salt, and pepper. Thinly slice lemons
and place on top of chicken.

4   Roast for 30 minutes or until vegetables are
tender and juices run clear when chicken is
pierced with tip of knife.

EACH SERVING: ABOUT 455 CALORIES, 53G PROTEIN,
19G CARBOHYDRATE, 18G TOTAL FAT (4G SATURATED),
6G FIBER, 231MG CHOLESTEROL, 805MG SODIUM.

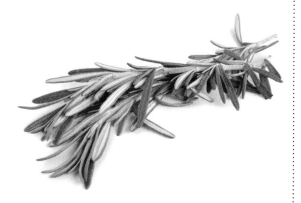

CHICKEN WITH
Orange Relish

Chicken is roasted with fresh ginger, then topped
with a combo of cooked and fresh orange sections, more fresh
ginger, crunchy chopped celery, and chopped cilantro.

ACTIVE TIME: 15 MINUTES   TOTAL TIME: 25 MINUTES
MAKES: 4 MAIN-DISH SERVINGS

- 4   boneless, skinless chicken breast cutlets (4 ounces each)
- ¾   teaspoon grated, peeled fresh ginger
- ¼   teaspoon salt
- ¼   teaspoon ground black pepper
- 1   large navel orange
- 3   stalks celery, finely chopped
- 2   green onions, sliced
- 1   tablespoon red wine vinegar
- ¼   cup packed fresh cilantro leaves, finely chopped

1 Preheat oven to 425°F. Spray jelly-roll pan with nonstick cooking spray. Arrange chicken on pan. Rub chicken with ½ teaspoon ginger; sprinkle with ⅛ teaspoon salt and pepper. Roast for 10 to 12 minutes or until juices run clear when chicken is pierced with tip of knife.

2 Meanwhile, with knife, cut peel and white pith from orange; discard. Cut on either side of membrane to remove each section from orange; place half of sections in 2-quart saucepan. Squeeze juice from membranes into saucepan.

3 To same saucepan, add celery, onions, vinegar, remaining ¼ teaspoon ginger, and remaining ⅛ teaspoon salt. Heat to boiling over high heat. Reduce heat to simmer; cook, stirring occasionally, for 7 minutes or until celery is tender-crisp. Remove pan from heat; stir in cilantro and reserved orange sections.

4 Serve chicken with relish.

EACH SERVING: ABOUT 152 CALORIES, 24G PROTEIN, 7G CARBOHYDRATE, 3G TOTAL FAT (1G SATURATED), 2G FIBER, 63MG CHOLESTEROL, 205MG SODIUM.

> **TIP**
>
> You can also make this refreshing relish with 2 blood oranges.

CHICKEN WITH
Tex-Mex Salsa

What's our secret to a fabulous salsa using canned tomatoes? Start with the fire-roasted variety, then add a grilled jalapeño chile and garlic.

ACTIVE TIME: 20 MINUTES   **TOTAL TIME:** 30 MINUTES
MAKES: 4 MAIN-DISH SERVINGS

- ½ cup finely chopped white onion
- 1 jalapeño chile
- 3 garlic cloves
- 1 can (14½ ounces) fire-roasted diced tomatoes, drained well
- ¼ cup packed fresh cilantro leaves, chopped
- 1 tablespoon fresh lime juice
- 1 teaspoon salt
- ½ teaspoon ground black pepper
- 1 cut-up chicken (3 to 3½ pounds), 8 pieces total

1 Prepare outdoor grill for covered direct grilling over medium heat.

2 Prepare salsa: In small bowl, soak onion in *cold water*. Wrap jalapeño and garlic in foil. Place foil packet on hot grill rack. Cook for 17 minutes or until vegetables are charred and blackened in spots; cool. Remove stem, skin, and seeds from jalapeño. Peel garlic; chop. Transfer to food processor with knife blade attached, along with tomatoes, cilantro, lime juice, and ½ teaspoon salt. Pulse until finely chopped. Drain onion and stir into mixture.

3 Sprinkle remaining ½ teaspoon salt and pepper all over chicken. Place on hot grill rack, skin-side down. Cover and cook for 15 to 20 minutes or until juices run clear when chicken is pierced with tip of knife, turning over once. (Smaller pieces will cook more quickly.)

4 Serve chicken with salsa.

EACH SERVING: ABOUT 425 CALORIES, 43G PROTEIN, 7G CARBOHYDRATE, 24G TOTAL FAT (7G SATURATED), 1G FIBER, 134MG CHOLESTEROL, 870MG SODIUM.

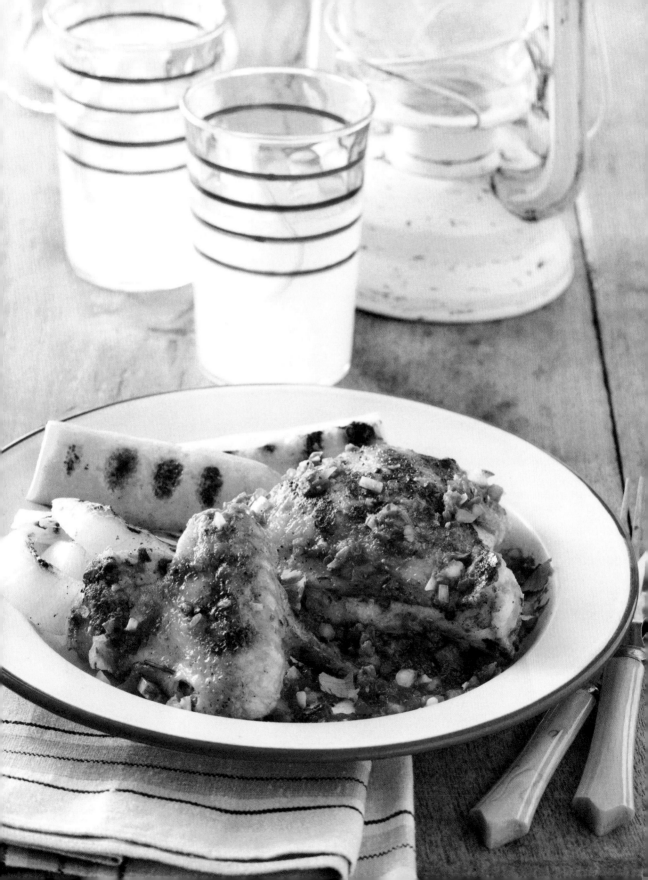

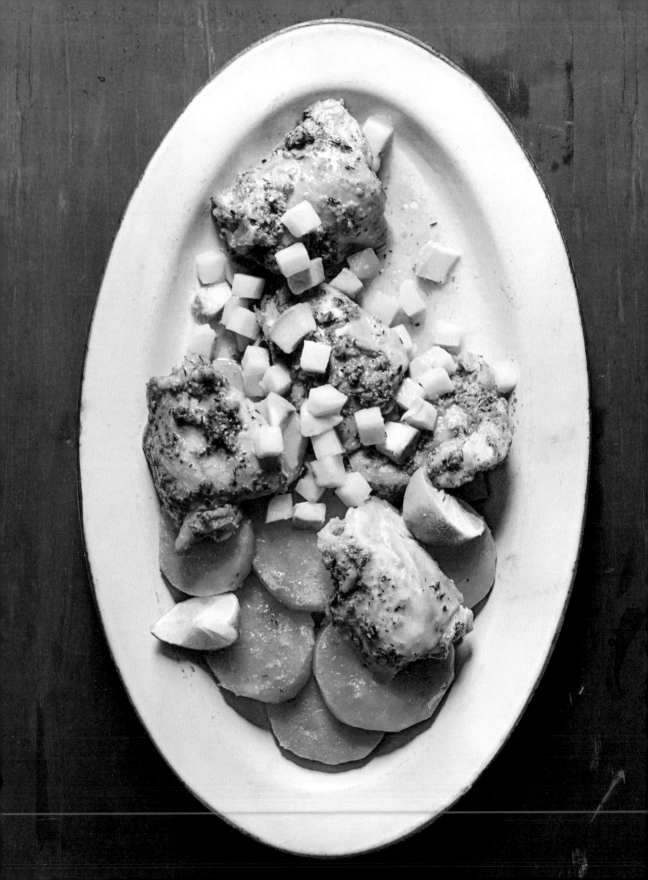

Caribbean
CHICKEN THIGHS

Chicken slow-cooked with sweet potatoes, orange juice,
jalapeño, cumin, and thyme is then topped with
a creamy mango and avocado salsa.

ACTIVE TIME: 20 MINUTES   **TOTAL TIME:** 4 HOURS 20 MINUTES
MAKES: 4 MAIN-DISH SERVINGS

2   large sweet potatoes, peeled and sliced into
    ½-inch-thick rounds

¼   cup no-pulp orange juice

¼   cup Rich Chicken Broth (page 14) or lower-
    sodium chicken broth

Salt

5   garlic cloves

1   jalapeño chile, chopped

2   tablespoons olive oil

2   tablespoons ground cumin

1   teaspoon dried thyme

3   pounds bone-in skinless chicken thighs

1   mango, cubed

1   avocado, cubed

1   tablespoon fresh lime juice

1 In 6- to 6½-quart slow-cooker bowl, layer sweet potatoes. Mix orange juice, broth, and ¼ teaspoon salt in bowl; pour over potatoes.

2 In food processor with knife blade attached, blend garlic, jalapeño, oil, cumin, and thyme into smooth paste.

3 Sprinkle chicken with ¼ teaspoon salt. Arrange over potatoes; spread with garlic mixture. Cover slow cooker and cook on high for 4 hours or on low for 8 hours.

4 About 5 minutes before serving, in bowl, toss mango, avocado, lime juice, and pinch salt.

5 Serve chicken with sweet potatoes topped with salsa.

EACH SERVING: ABOUT 595 CALORIES, 44G PROTEIN, 39G CARBOHYDRATE, 24G TOTAL FAT (4G SATURATED), 10G FIBER, 213MG CHOLESTEROL, 554MG SODIUM.

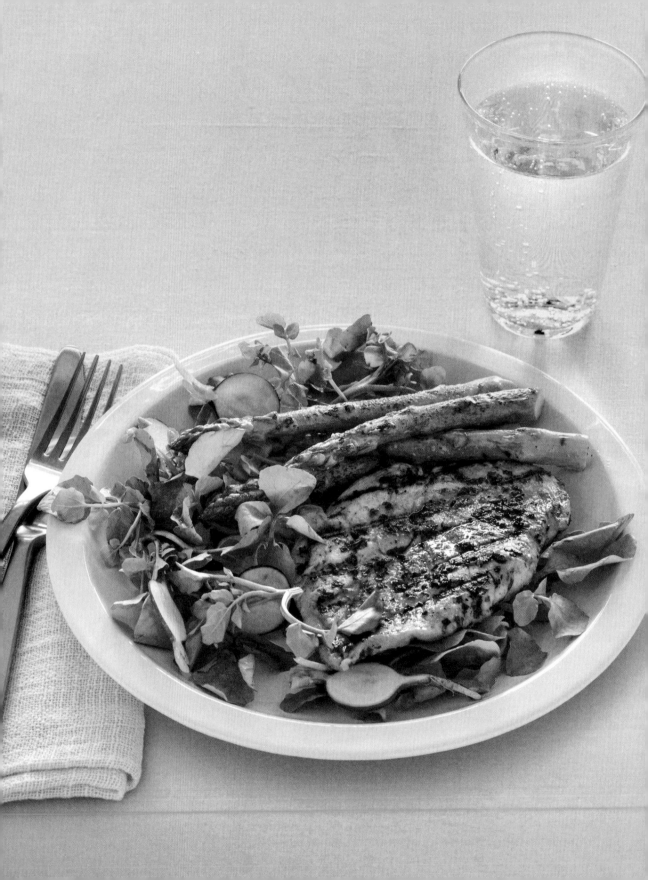

GRILLED
Chicken & Greens

This lemony-mint chicken with asparagus
and radishes makes the perfect springtime meal.

ACTIVE TIME: 20 MINUTES **TOTAL TIME:** 30 MINUTES
MAKES: 4 MAIN-DISH SERVINGS

1 pound boneless, skinless chicken breast
  halves

1 cup packed fresh mint leaves

1 lemon

2 garlic cloves, crushed with press

1 tablespoon plus 2 teaspoons extra-virgin
  olive oil

Salt and ground black pepper

1 pound asparagus, ends trimmed

1 pound radishes, trimmed and very
  thinly sliced

2 packages (4 ounces each) watercress

1 Prepare outdoor grill for direct grilling over
medium-high heat, or preheat large ridged grill
pan over medium-high heat.

2 With meat mallet, pound chicken (placed
between two sheets of plastic wrap) to an even
$\frac{1}{3}$-inch thickness.

3 Finely chop half of mint. From lemon, finely
grate 1 teaspoon peel and squeeze 4 tablespoons
juice. In 9-inch pie plate, combine chopped
mint, lemon peel, 1 tablespoon lemon juice,

half of garlic, 1 teaspoon oil, and $\frac{1}{8}$ teaspoon
each salt and pepper. Add chicken and rub with
mint mixture to evenly coat.

4 On jelly-roll pan, toss asparagus with
1 teaspoon oil, pinch each salt and pepper, and
remaining garlic. Place asparagus on hot grill
rack. Cook for 4 to 6 minutes or until charred
in spots, turning occasionally.

5 Meanwhile, in large bowl, toss radishes,
watercress, 3 tablespoons lemon juice,
1 tablespoon oil, $\frac{1}{8}$ teaspoon each salt and
pepper, and remaining mint. Divide among
four plates. Place hot asparagus on top of greens.

6 Place chicken on hot grill rack. Cook for 4
to 6 minutes or until browned and no longer
pink throughout, turning over once. Divide hot
chicken among plates with greens.

EACH SERVING: ABOUT 225 CALORIES, 27G PROTEIN,
10G CARBOHYDRATE, 9G TOTAL FAT (2G SATURATED),
5G FIBER, 63MG CHOLESTEROL, 315MG SODIUM.

Caramelized Cauliflower & Green Olives

Roasting cauliflower is a great way to bring out its natural sweetness. We pair it with quick-cooking chicken tenders and then toss everything in a savory green sauce with olives and almonds.

ACTIVE TIME: 10 MINUTES   **TOTAL TIME:** 50 MINUTES
MAKES: 4 MAIN-DISH SERVINGS

1   head cauliflower (2½ to 3 pounds), trimmed and cut into 1½-inch chunks

2   tablespoons extra-virgin olive oil

Salt and ground black pepper

1½ pounds chicken breast tenders, cut into 1½-inch chunks

1   teaspoon freshly grated lemon peel

¼   cup slivered almonds

⅓   cup pitted green olives, rinsed well

¼   cup packed fresh flat-leaf parsley, finely chopped, plus additional for garnish

1 Preheat oven to 450°F. In 18" by 12" jelly-roll pan, combine cauliflower, 2 teaspoons oil, and ⅛ teaspoon each salt and pepper until well mixed. Spread cauliflower in single layer on pan. Roast for 20 to 25 minutes or until cauliflower is golden brown.

2 While cauliflower roasts, in large bowl, combine chicken, lemon peel, 1 teaspoon oil, and ¼ teaspoon each salt and pepper. Push cauliflower to one side of pan and arrange chicken in single layer on other side. Roast for 10 minutes more or until chicken just loses its pink color throughout.

3 Meanwhile, in food processor with knife blade attached, pulse almonds until finely ground. Add olives and parsley and pulse until almost smooth. With machine running, add remaining 1 tablespoon oil until fully incorporated, scraping sides of bowl as needed. Add mixture to pan with hot chicken and cauliflower and stir until well combined. Transfer to serving plates and garnish with additional parsley.

EACH SERVING: ABOUT 360 CALORIES, 45G PROTEIN, 12G CARBOHYDRATE, 15G TOTAL FAT (2G SATURATED), 6G FIBER, 99MG CHOLESTEROL, 660MG SODIUM.

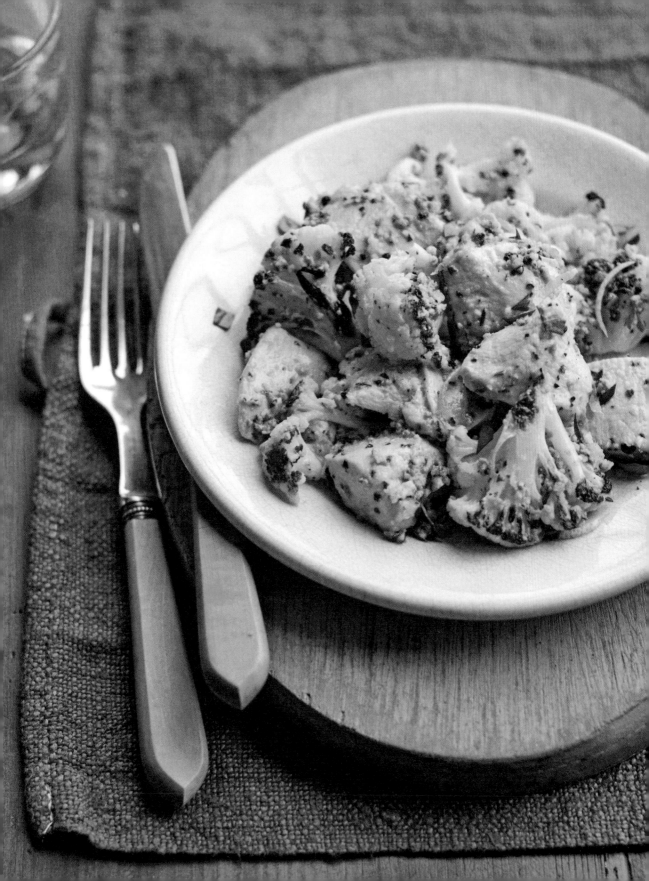

GRILLED CHICKEN WITH
Vegetables & Avocado Salsa

Grilled chicken breasts, bell peppers, and tomatoes
are slathered with lime and topped
with a crunchy avocado and jicama salsa.

ACTIVE TIME: 20 MINUTES   **TOTAL TIME:** 30 MINUTES
MAKES: 4 MAIN-DISH SERVINGS

4   boneless, skinless chicken breast halves
    (6 ounces each)

¾   teaspoon salt

¼   teaspoon ground black pepper

1   lime

2   tablespoons olive or avocado oil

2   tomatoes (10 ounces each), cut crosswise into
    ½-inch-thick slices

2   red, orange, and/or yellow peppers (4 to
    6 ounces each), cut into quarters

1   ripe avocado, cut into ½-inch chunks

1   cup chopped jicama

¼   cup loosely packed fresh cilantro leaves,
    chopped, plus additional leaves for garnish

⅛   teaspoon cayenne (ground red) pepper

1 Prepare outdoor grill for direct grilling over medium heat, or preheat large ridged grill pan over medium heat.

2 Meanwhile, place chicken, 1 breast at a time, between two sheets of plastic wrap. With meat mallet, rolling pin, or heavy skillet, pound two or three times to an even ½-inch thickness. Sprinkle chicken evenly with ¼ teaspoon salt and ⅛ teaspoon pepper.

3 From lime, grate 1½ teaspoons peel and squeeze 3 tablespoons juice. In small bowl, combine peel, 1 tablespoon juice, oil, ¼ teaspoon salt, and remaining ⅛ teaspoon pepper.

4 Brush tomatoes and peppers with oil mixture. Place vegetables on hot grill rack. Cook for 8 to 9 minutes or until browned and tender, turning over once. Place chicken on hot grill rack. Cook for 8 to 9 minutes or until browned on both sides and no longer pink throughout, turning over once.

5 While vegetables and chicken are grilling, in medium bowl, combine avocado, jicama, chopped cilantro, cayenne, remaining ¼ teaspoon salt, and remaining 2 tablespoons lime juice. Stir. Makes 2½ cups salsa.

6 Serve chicken and vegetables with avocado salsa; garnish with cilantro leaves.

EACH SERVING: ABOUT 380 CALORIES, 42G PROTEIN, 17G CARBOHYDRATE, 17G TOTAL FAT (3G SATURATED), 7G FIBER, 99MG CHOLESTEROL, 545MG SODIUM.

Salt-Free Rubs

Need more paleo-friendly chicken ideas? Add a zesty rub—this trio doesn't require added salt to taste great. To use, pat boneless, skinless chicken breast halves or thighs with paper towels. Sprinkle chicken with just enough rub to coat lightly (about 1 tablespoon per pound), and then grill, broil, or sauté. (Bonus: The zesty rubs can be made ahead and stored in airtight containers at room temperature for up to 6 months. They're excellent on meat and fish, too.)

HERB RUB

In small bowl, combine **2 tablespoons dried rosemary**, crumbled; **2 tablespoons dried thyme; 1 tablespoon dried tarragon;** and **1 tablespoon coarsely ground black pepper**.
Makes ⅔ cup.

SPICY PEPPERCORN RUB

In self-sealing plastic bag, combine **3 tablespoons coriander seeds, 3 tablespoons cumin seeds, 3 tablespoons fennel seeds,** and **1 tablespoon whole black peppercorns**. Place kitchen towel over bag and, with meat mallet or rolling pin, coarsely crush spices. Makes ⅓ cup.

RED CHILE RUB

In small bowl, combine **1 tablespoon dried cumin, 1 tablespoon paprika, 2 teaspoons ground chipotle chile pepper,** and **1 teaspoon dried oregano**.
Makes ¼ cup.

Coconut-Curry
CHICKEN

Coconut milk is a paleo go-to when you're
hankering for a rich and creamy dish without the dairy.

ACTIVE TIME: 20 MINUTES · **TOTAL TIME:** 35 MINUTES
MAKES: 2 MAIN-DISH SERVINGS

3   teaspoons coconut oil

12 ounces boneless, skinless chicken breast
    halves, cut into 1-inch chunks

½   teaspoon salt

1   medium onion (6 to 8 ounces), thinly sliced

1   medium red pepper (6 to 8 ounces), thinly
    sliced

1½ teaspoons minced jalapeño chile (from about
    ½ chile)

2   teaspoons fresh ginger, peeled and grated

2   garlic cloves, crushed with press

½   teaspoon curry powder

¾   cup light coconut milk

2   tablespoons packed fresh cilantro leaves,
    chopped

1 In 10-inch skillet, heat 2 teaspoons oil over
medium-high heat until hot. Sprinkle chicken
with ¼ teaspoon salt; add to skillet and cook,
stirring occasionally, for 3 to 4 minutes or until
golden. Transfer chicken to plate.

2 In same skillet, heat remaining 1 teaspoon
oil over medium heat until hot. Add onion and
cook, stirring occasionally, for 3 minutes or
until softened. Stir in pepper, jalapeño, ginger,
and garlic; cook, stirring, for 1 minute or until
fragrant. Stir in curry powder; cook for 1 minute.
Stir in coconut milk, stirring until browned bits
are loosened from bottom of pan.

3 Return chicken to skillet and cook for 3 to 5
minutes or just until chicken is no longer pink
throughout. Remove skillet from heat and stir in
cilantro and remaining ¼ teaspoon salt.

EACH SERVING: ABOUT 393 CALORIES, 42G PROTEIN,
17G CARBOHYDRATE, 17G TOTAL FAT (12G SATURATED),
4G FIBER, 124MG CHOLESTEROL, 584MG SODIUM.

TIP
Just before serving, sprinkle the curry with
fresh cilantro leaves, golden raisins, and
sliced toasted almonds.

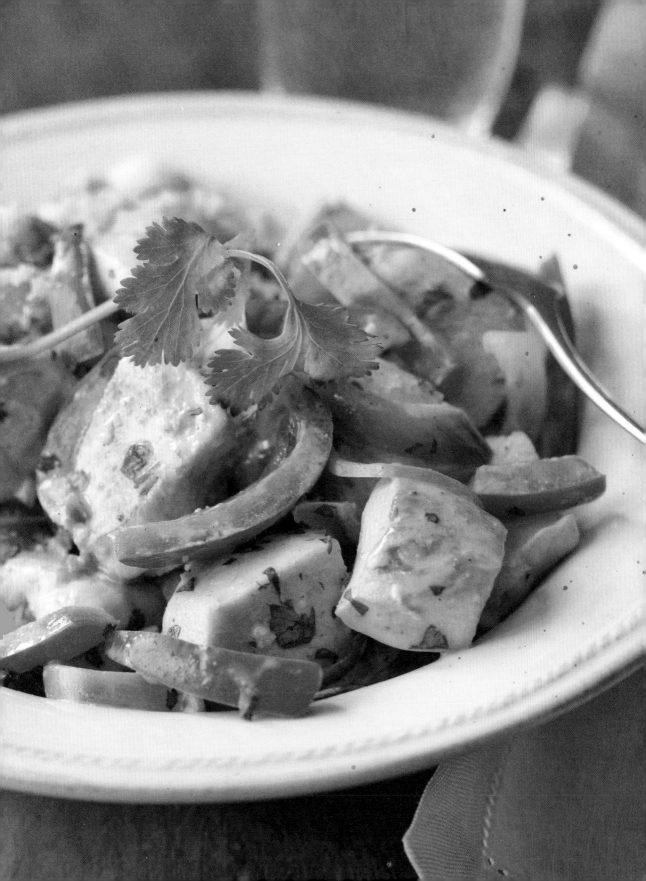

Tarragon Turkey
WITH GRAPES

Seedless grapes are an unexpected but delicious addition to savory dishes. Their mild sweetness also complements the flavor of quick-cooking turkey cutlets.

ACTIVE TIME: 15 MINUTES   **TOTAL TIME:** 30 MINUTES
MAKES: 4 MAIN-DISH SERVINGS

- 4 turkey cutlets (6 ounces each)
- 3 teaspoons chopped fresh tarragon leaves, plus additional sprigs for garnish
- ¼ teaspoon salt
- ¼ teaspoon ground black pepper
- 4 teaspoons olive oil
- 1 small onion (4 to 6 ounces), chopped
- ½ cup dry white wine
- 2 cups seedless red grapes
- 1 cup Rich Chicken Broth (page 14) or lower-sodium chicken broth

1 Sprinkle turkey with 2 teaspoons chopped tarragon, salt, and pepper.

2 In 12-inch skillet, heat 2 teaspoons oil over medium heat until hot. Add turkey and cook for 12 to 14 minutes or until browned and no longer pink throughout, turning over once. Transfer turkey to platter; cover with foil to keep warm.

3 To same skillet, add remaining 2 teaspoons oil and heat over medium heat until hot. Add onion and cook, stirring occasionally, for 6 minutes or until tender. Stir in wine; increase heat to medium-high and cook for 1 minute. Add grapes, broth, and remaining 1 teaspoon tarragon and heat to boiling. Cook, stirring occasionally, for 5 minutes or until grapes are tender.

4 To serve, spoon grape sauce over turkey and garnish with tarragon sprigs.

EACH SERVING: ABOUT 306 CALORIES, 41G PROTEIN, 18G CARBOHYDRATE, 7G TOTAL FAT (1G SATURATED), 1G FIBER, 97MG CHOLESTEROL, 423MG SODIUM.

"SPAGHETTI" WITH
Turkey Bolognese

You won't miss the pasta in this hearty dish
featuring spaghetti squash and a speedy tomato sauce.
Top each serving with chopped fresh basil, if you wish.

ACTIVE TIME: 15 MINUTES   **TOTAL TIME:** 35 MINUTES
MAKES: 4 MAIN-DISH SERVINGS

2   small spaghetti squash (2½ pounds each)

1   tablespoon olive oil

1   medium onion, chopped

1   medium red pepper, chopped

3   garlic cloves, minced

½   teaspoon salt

12 ounces lean ground turkey

1   can (28 ounces) crushed tomatoes

¼   teaspoon ground black pepper

1 With small knife, pierce each squash all over. On microwave-safe plate, microwave squash on High for 15 minutes.

2 Meanwhile, in large saucepot, heat oil over medium-high heat until hot. Add onion, red pepper, garlic, and salt. Cook, stirring often, for 10 minutes or until vegetables are tender. Add turkey and cook for 5 minutes or until browned, breaking up meat with side of spoon. Add tomatoes and simmer for 10 minutes or until flavors are blended. Stir in pepper.

3 Cut each squash in half lengthwise; scoop out seeds and discard. With two forks, scrape out pulp from squash. Serve sauce over each squash half.

EACH SERVING: ABOUT 370 CALORIES, 23G PROTEIN, 47G CARBOHYDRATE, 13G TOTAL FAT (3G SATURATED), 11G FIBER, 63MG CHOLESTEROL, 745MG SODIUM.

Salmon with Gingery Cabbage (page 86)

5 | Fabulous Fish & Shellfish

Make the catch of the day your dinner tonight! Seafood lovers will dive into our Scallop & Cherry Tomato Skewers and Fisherman's Stew. Or, if salmon is your fish of choice, our Ginger-Crusted Salmon with Melon Salsa and Salmon Steaks with Tricolor Pepper Relish are hard to beat. As for other fish, we offer delicious recipes like Jerk Halibut with Apple-Sweet Potato Mash and Roasted Cod & Mushroom Ragout. Pair that with our foolproof cooking tips and you'll have all the goods necessary for a deep-sea adventure in the kitchen.

SALMON WITH
Gingery Cabbage

We pair curry mustard-roasted salmon
with sautéed cabbage, fresh ginger, and ground cumin.
For photo, see page 84.

ACTIVE TIME: 10 MINUTES   **TOTAL TIME:** 20 MINUTES
MAKES: 4 MAIN-DISH SERVINGS

1 tablespoon olive oil

1 small onion, thinly sliced

4 pieces salmon fillet (6 ounces each), skin removed

½ teaspoon curry powder

2 tablespoons Dijon mustard with seeds

2 teaspoons grated, peeled fresh ginger

½ teaspoon ground cumin

1 bag (16 ounces) shredded cabbage for coleslaw

¼ teaspoon salt

1 Preheat oven to 400°F. In 12-inch nonstick skillet, heat oil over medium heat until hot. Add onion; cover and cook, stirring occasionally, for 8 to 10 minutes or until tender and golden brown.

2 Meanwhile, grease 13" by 9" glass baking dish. Place salmon, rounded-sides up, in baking dish. In cup, stir together curry powder, mustard, and *2 teaspoons water*; brush evenly over salmon.

3 Roast salmon, without turning over, for 15 minutes or until just opaque throughout.

4 While salmon roasts, add ginger and cumin to onion in skillet. Cook, stirring, for 1 minute or until fragrant. Add cabbage and salt; cover and cook, stirring occasionally, for 11 to 13 minutes or until cabbage is just tender and starts to brown.

5 To serve, spoon cabbage mixture onto four dinner plates; top with salmon.

EACH SERVING: ABOUT 250 CALORIES, 31G PROTEIN, 6G CARBOHYDRATE, 11G TOTAL FAT (2G SATURATED), 2G FIBER, 73MG CHOLESTEROL, 450MG SODIUM.

Sustainable Seafood

If you love fish but are concerned about its supply and environmental impact, then it's important to learn about sustainable seafood. Simply defined, seafood is sustainable when the population of a fish species is managed to meet market demands without damaging the ability of that species to reproduce and remain available for future generations. What are the best sustainable seafood choices?

First step, buy U.S. fish. The U.S. has strict environmental and food safety laws governing farmed and wild-caught fish. For specific fish, here are the latest recommendations from the NOAA Fisheries Service (the U.S. authority on marine fisheries science, conservation, and management) and the Monterey Bay Aquarium:

VARIETY	TYPE
Clams	Farm-raised hard clams (aka: quahog, round clam, chowder clam)
Cod	Wild-caught Pacific cod and Atlantic cod
Crab	Wild-caught red king (Alaskan king) crab and Alaskan snow crab
Flounder	Wild-caught arrowtooth, summer flounder (fluke), and yellowtail flounder
Halibut	Wild-caught Pacific (Alaskan) halibut
Mussels	Farm-raised blue mussels
Oysters	Farm-raised Eastern or Pacific oysters
Salmon	Wild-caught or farm-raised Atlantic salmon; wild-caught coho salmon
Scallops	Wild-caught Atlantic scallops
Shrimp	Wild-caught shrimp
Sole	Wild-caught sole
Striped Bass	Wild-caught Atlantic striped bass (rockfish)
Tuna	Wild-caught Pacific bluefin tuna and western Atlantic bluefin tuna

SEARED SALMON
with Sweet Potatoes

A complete fish dinner in 30 minutes?
Yes—when you micro-steam the potatoes.

ACTIVE TIME: 15 MINUTES **TOTAL TIME:** 30 MINUTES
MAKES: 4 MAIN-DISH SERVINGS

- 1 pound sweet potatoes, peeled and cut into ½-inch cubes
- Salt
- ¼ teaspoon ground black pepper
- 1 teaspoon olive oil
- 1 bag (6 ounces) baby spinach
- ⅛ teaspoon cayenne (ground red) pepper
- 4 pieces center-cut salmon fillet (5 ounces each), skin removed
- 1 lemon
- 1 cup dry white wine
- 2 teaspoons capers, rinsed
- ¼ cup fresh flat-leaf parsley leaves, chopped

1 In large microwave-safe bowl, combine potatoes, ¼ *cup water*, ¼ teaspoon salt, and pepper. Cover with vented plastic wrap; microwave on high for 9 minutes or until tender, stirring halfway through cooking. Add spinach; re-cover and microwave for 2 minutes more.

2 Meanwhile, sprinkle salmon with cayenne and ⅛ teaspoon salt. In 12-inch nonstick skillet, heat oil over medium heat until hot. Add salmon and cook for 10 minutes or until just opaque throughout, turning over halfway through cooking. Transfer to plate. From lemon, finely grate ½ teaspoon peel onto fish; into cup, squeeze 1 tablespoon juice.

3 To skillet, add wine and capers. Boil over high heat for 2 minutes or until liquid is reduced by half, stirring until browned bits are loosened from bottom of pan. Remove from heat; stir in lemon juice and parsley.

4 Divide potato mixture among plates; top with fish. Spoon sauce over fish.

EACH SERVING: ABOUT 300 CALORIES, 31G PROTEIN, 22G CARBOHYDRATE, 9G TOTAL FAT (1G SATURATED), 4G FIBER, 78MG CHOLESTEROL, 430MG SODIUM.

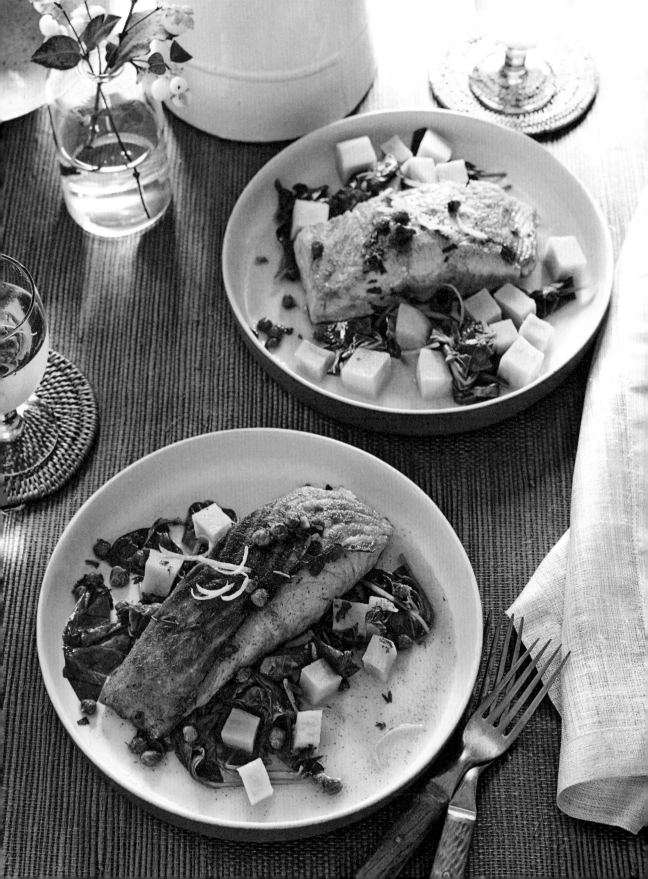

SALMON STEAKS WITH
Tricolor Pepper Relish

Salmon steaks are a great bargain.
The tasty relish is a combo of roasted peppers,
fresh basil, sun-dried tomatoes, and capers.

ACTIVE TIME: 15 MINUTES **TOTAL TIME:** 45 MINUTES
MAKES: 4 MAIN-DISH SERVINGS

¼ cup sliced almonds

3 medium peppers (4 to 6 ounces each), preferably red, yellow, and orange, thinly sliced

1 small onion (4 to 6 ounces), thinly sliced

1 tablespoon olive oil

Salt and ground black pepper

2 salmon steaks (12 to 14 ounces each)

½ cup packed fresh basil leaves, finely chopped, plus additional for garnish

¼ cup oil-packed sun-dried tomatoes, patted dry and chopped

1 tablespoon capers, coarsely chopped

1 Preheat oven to 450°F. In 18" by 12" jelly-roll pan, spread almonds in single layer. Roast for 4 to 6 minutes or until toasted. Transfer to plate; set aside. In same pan, combine peppers, onion, oil, and ⅛ teaspoon each salt and pepper. Spread in single layer; roast for 15 minutes or until tender. Stir vegetables; push to one side of pan to make space for salmon.

2 Sprinkle salmon with ¼ teaspoon each salt and pepper to season both sides. Place in pan with peppers. Roast for 8 to 10 minutes or until salmon is just opaque throughout and a knife pierces easily through flesh.

3 Meanwhile, in large bowl, combine basil, tomatoes, and capers. Add roasted peppers and onion and stir well. Cut each salmon steak lengthwise in half; remove and discard bones. Divide salmon among serving plates and top with pepper relish and almonds.

....

EACH SERVING: ABOUT 395 CALORIES, 40G PROTEIN, 14G CARBOHYDRATE, 20G TOTAL FAT (3G SATURATED), 4G FIBER, 101MG CHOLESTEROL, 385MG SODIUM.

TIP

If fresh basil is not in season, substitute an equal amount of flat-leaf parsley.

Fish & Pesto

Are you a newbie at cooking fish? Want to up your seafood smarts?
Follow these handy hints for perfect "net results" every time, then grab
your blender and whip up a fabulous, fish-friendly pesto.

SKIP FLIPPING FISH Buy ½-inch-thick (or less) fish fillets or steaks. Cook on one side.

THICK PIECES OF FISH Follow the 10 Minute Rule: Cook fish for 10 minutes per inch, turning over once with a spatula.

ODOR-EATERS To help cook fish without the smell, place a cup of vinegar nearby to absorb the odors, or light a scented candle 10 minutes before getting started.

EXTRA-MOIST WHOLE FISH Don't be tempted to remove the head or tail before cooking, as they help the fish stay moist. Instead, remove the head and tail from cooked fish before serving, if desired.

BETTER-BAKED FISH If fish has a topping or is brushed with oil, make several shallow cuts in the flesh before baking. This will help the flavors permeate and keep the fish moist.

. . . .

SICILIAN PESTO

Blend **1 cup sun-dried tomatoes packed in oil**, drained; **½ cup olive oil**; **¼ cup packed fresh parsley**; **2 tablespoons fresh lemon juice**; **1 tablespoon capers**, drained; **1 teaspoon freshly grated lemon peel**; and **1 garlic clove** until mostly smooth.

. . . .

SPICY THAI PESTO

Blend **1 medium sweet long red pepper**, seeded and chopped; **½ cup olive oil**; **1 stalk lemongrass**, outer layer discarded and thinly sliced; **2 thin slices ginger**; **2 Thai chiles** (or 2 serrano chiles); **2 tablespoons Asian fish sauce**; **1 garlic clove**; and **½ teaspoon coriander seeds** until smooth.

. . . .

PEPITA PESTO

Blend **1 cup packed fresh cilantro leaves**, **½ cup olive or avocado oil**, **⅓ cup pumpkin seeds** (pepitas), **2 tablespoons fresh lime juice**, **1 garlic clove**, **¼ teaspoon cayenne (ground red) pepper**, and **½ teaspoon salt** until mostly smooth.

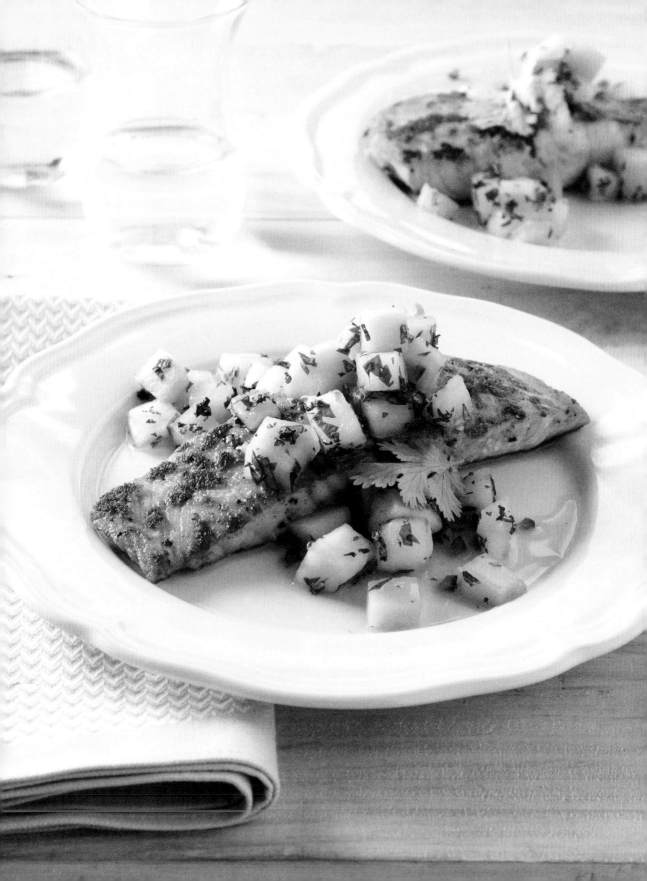

GINGER-CRUSTED SALMON
with Melon Salsa

A refreshing melon-mint salsa is the
perfect complement to the rich taste of salmon.

ACTIVE TIME: 20 MINUTES   **TOTAL TIME:** 35 MINUTES

MAKES: 4 MAIN-DISH SERVINGS

2   cups cubed cantaloupe (⅓-inch pieces)

1   cup cubed honeydew (⅓-inch pieces)

¼   cup packed fresh cilantro leaves, finely
    chopped

2   tablespoons fresh mint leaves, finely
    chopped

1   jalapeño chile, seeded and finely chopped

2   tablespoons fresh lime juice

Salt

½   teaspoon ground black pepper

2   tablespoons grated, peeled fresh ginger

2   teaspoons curry powder

4   pieces salmon fillet (6 ounces each), skin
    removed

2   teaspoons olive oil

1 In medium bowl, combine cantaloupe, honeydew, cilantro, mint, jalapeño, lime juice, and ¼ teaspoon salt and stir until well mixed; set aside.

2 In small bowl, combine ginger, curry powder, ⅛ teaspoon salt, and pepper. Spread mixture evenly over skinless side of each fillet.

3 In 12-inch nonstick skillet, heat oil over medium heat for 1 minute or until hot. Add salmon, ginger-side down, and cook for 10 minutes or until salmon is just opaque throughout, turning over once. Serve salmon with melon salsa.

EACH SERVING: ABOUT 350 CALORIES, 40G PROTEIN, 13G CARBOHYDRATE, 15G TOTAL FAT (2G SATURATED), 2G FIBER, 108MG CHOLESTEROL, 325MG SODIUM.

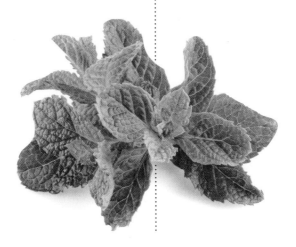

COD
Livornese

The Tuscan seaport town of Livorno is
famous for this simple preparation of white fish featuring
Mediterranean favorites: tomatoes, olives, and capers.

ACTIVE TIME: 15 MINUTES **TOTAL TIME:** 30 MINUTES
MAKES: 4 MAIN-DISH SERVINGS

1 tablespoon chopped fresh oregano leaves

2 teaspoons freshly grated lemon peel

2 teaspoons plus 2 tablespoons olive oil

¼ teaspoon salt

4 pieces cod fillet (6 ounces each)

1 pint cherry tomatoes

¼ cup Kalamata olives

2 tablespoons capers, drained

⅛ teaspoon crushed red pepper

2 garlic cloves, minced

¼ cup loosely packed fresh parsley leaves, chopped

1 In cup, combine oregano, lemon peel, 2 teaspoons oil, and salt. Rub both sides of cod fillets with oregano mixture.

2 In 12-inch nonstick skillet, heat 1 tablespoon oil over medium heat until hot. Add cod and cook for 8 to 10 minutes or until fish is just opaque throughout, turning over once. Transfer cod to four dinner plates.

3 In same skillet, heat remaining 1 tablespoon oil over medium heat until hot. Stir in tomatoes, olives, capers, crushed red pepper, and garlic; cook, stirring occasionally, for 6 to 8 minutes or just until tomatoes are heated through and skins split. Stir in parsley; serve with cod.

EACH SERVING: ABOUT 250 CALORIES, 31G PROTEIN, 6G CARBOHYDRATE, 11G TOTAL FAT (2G SATURATED), 2G FIBER, 73MG CHOLESTEROL, 450MG SODIUM.

TIP

This dish is also excellent with halibut fillets.

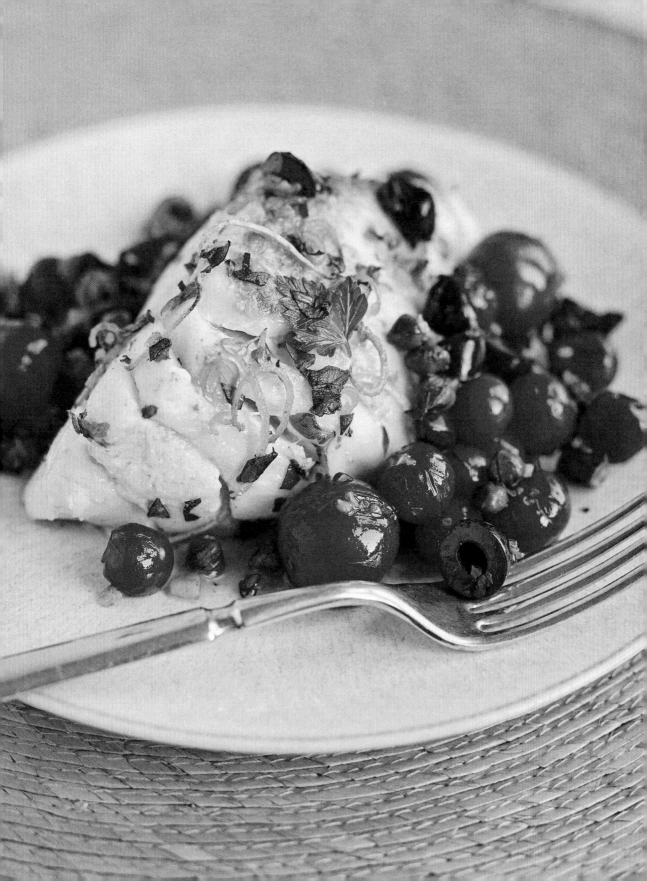

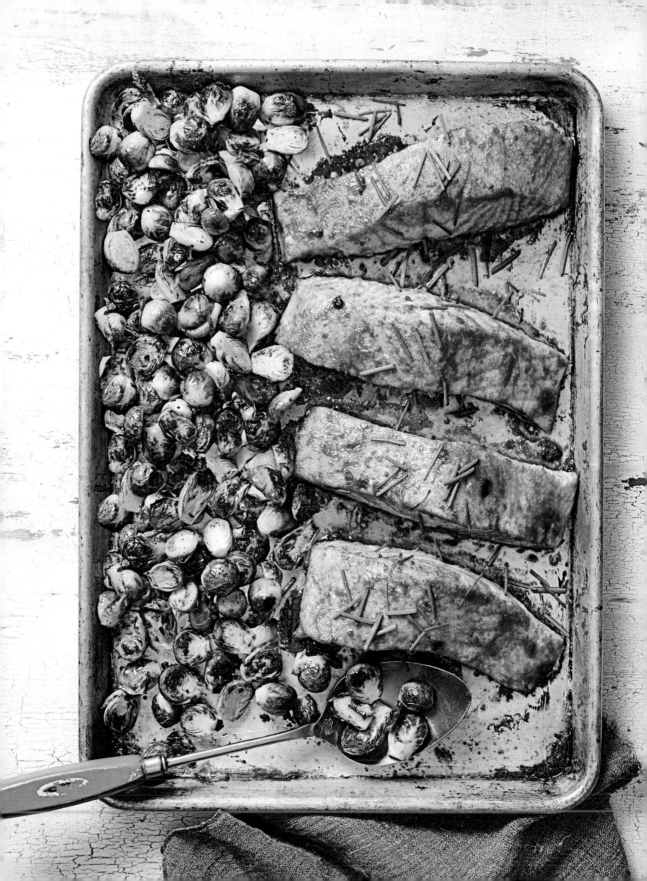

"BBQ" SALMON
& Brussels Bake

Unrefined sugar, like honey, can be an occasional treat on the paleo plan. When paired with smoked paprika, honey gives this dish its "barbecue" taste.

ACTIVE TIME: 20 MINUTES   **TOTAL TIME:** 40 MINUTES
MAKES: 6 MAIN-DISH SERVINGS

1½ tablespoons honey

1   teaspoon garlic powder

1   teaspoon onion powder

1   teaspoon smoked paprika

3   tablespoons olive oil

1¼ pounds Brussels sprouts, trimmed and halved

1¼ teaspoons salt

¼   teaspoon ground black pepper

1   side of salmon (about 3½ pounds)

Snipped chives, for garnish

1 Preheat oven to 450°F. Line large rimmed baking sheet with foil. In small bowl with wire whisk, mix honey, garlic powder, onion powder, smoked paprika, and 2 tablespoons oil until well blended.

2 On another large rimmed baking sheet, toss Brussels sprouts with remaining 1 tablespoon oil, ¼ teaspoon salt, and pepper. Roast sprouts for 5 minutes.

3 Meanwhile, cut salmon into 10 fillets; arrange skin-side down on prepared baking sheet. Brush rub all over salmon; sprinkle with remaining 1 teaspoon salt. Roast salmon with Brussels sprouts for 15 minutes or until sprouts are tender and salmon is just cooked through, stirring sprouts once halfway through roasting. Reserve 4 smaller salmon fillets for another use. Serve remaining salmon with Brussels sprouts and garnish with chives.

EACH SERVING: ABOUT 280 CALORIES, 35G PROTEIN, 11G CARBOHYDRATE, 11G TOTAL FAT (2G SATURATED), 3G FIBER, 74MG CHOLESTEROL, 379MG SODIUM.

ROASTED COD &
Mushroom Ragout

The rich earthiness of sweet potatoes and mushrooms blends perfectly with a delicate, mild-tasting fish like cod.

TOTAL TIME: 15 MINUTES **MAKES:** 4 MAIN-DISH SERVINGS

1 large sweet potato (1 pound), peeled and cut into ½-inch chunks

2 tablespoons extra-virgin olive oil

2 large shallots, thinly sliced

½ teaspoon salt

½ teaspoon ground black pepper

2 packages (10 ounces each) sliced mushrooms

4 cod fillets (6 ounces each)

¼ cup packed fresh flat-leaf parsley leaves, finely chopped

½ cup dry white wine

1 Preheat oven to 450°F.

2 On 18" by 12" jelly-roll pan, combine sweet potatoes, 1 tablespoon oil, half the shallots, and ⅛ teaspoon each salt and pepper. Arrange in single layer on one side of pan. Roast for 15 minutes.

3 Meanwhile, in 12-inch skillet, heat remaining 1 tablespoon oil over medium-high heat until hot. Add remaining shallots and cook, stirring occasionally, for 2 to 3 minutes or until tender and golden brown. Add mushrooms and *2 tablespoons water*; cook, stirring occasionally, for 8 minutes or until liquid evaporates.

4 Arrange cod on other side of roasting pan. Sprinkle with ⅛ teaspoon each salt and pepper. Roast alongside potatoes for 8 to 10 minutes or until fish is just opaque throughout.

5 Stir parsley, wine, and remaining ¼ teaspoon each salt and pepper into mushroom mixture. Cook for 1 minute or until wine is reduced by half.

6 Divide potatoes and cod among serving plates. Spoon mushroom ragout over cod.

EACH SERVING: ABOUT 295 CALORIES, 33G PROTEIN, 22G CARBOHYDRATE, 9G TOTAL FAT (1G SATURATED), 4G FIBER, 65MG CHOLESTEROL, 420MG SODIUM.

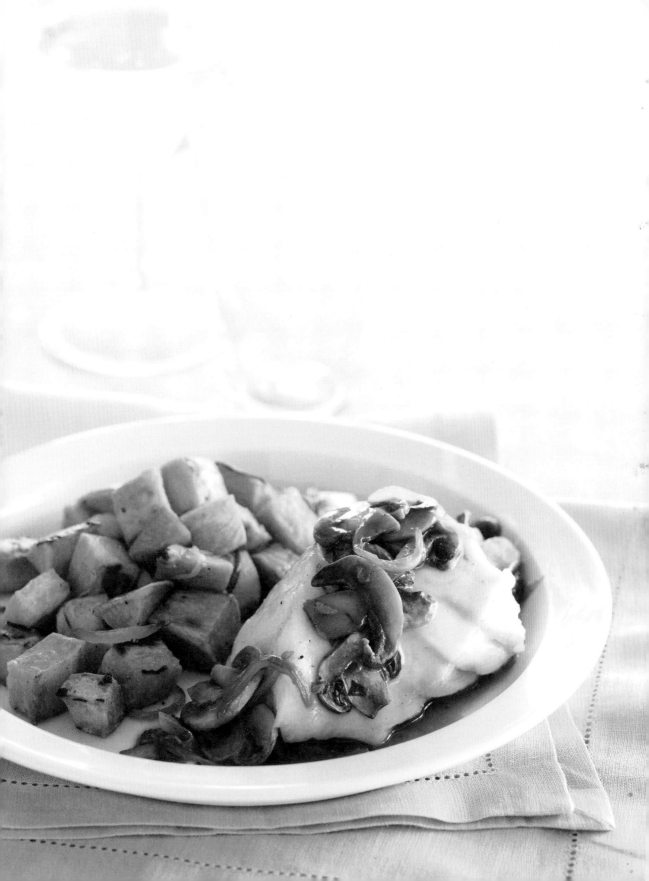

JERK HALIBUT WITH
Apple-Sweet Potato Mash

We recommend using salt-free jerk seasoning—the spice combination
is so flavorful, you won't even miss it.

TOTAL TIME: 15 MINUTES   **MAKES:** 4 MAIN-DISH SERVINGS

2   pounds sweet potatoes, peeled and cut into
    1-inch chunks

2   Granny Smith apples, peeled and cut into
    8 wedges

4   pieces halibut steak (6 ounces each), each
    1½ inches thick

1   tablespoon jerk seasoning

1   bag (9 ounces) microwave-in-bag broccoli
    florets

½   teaspoon salt

¼   teaspoon coarsely ground black pepper

1   lime, cut into 4 wedges

1 In 5- to 6-quart saucepot, place steamer basket
and *1 inch water*; heat to boiling over high heat.
Place potatoes and apples in steamer basket;
cover and steam over medium-low heat for 20
minutes or until potatoes and apples are tender.

2 Meanwhile, grease ridged grill pan; preheat
over medium heat. Rub both sides of halibut
steaks with jerk seasoning. Place halibut in hot
grill pan. Cook for 6 to 8 minutes or until just
opaque throughout, turning over once. While
halibut is cooking, microwave broccoli as
label directs.

3 Place potatoes and apples in large bowl; mash
with salt and pepper.

4 Serve halibut with lime wedges, mashed sweet
potatoes, and broccoli.

EACH SERVING: ABOUT 410 CALORIES, 40G PROTEIN,
53G CARBOHYDRATE, 5G TOTAL FAT (1G SATURATED),
8G FIBER, 54MG CHOLESTEROL, 630MG SODIUM.

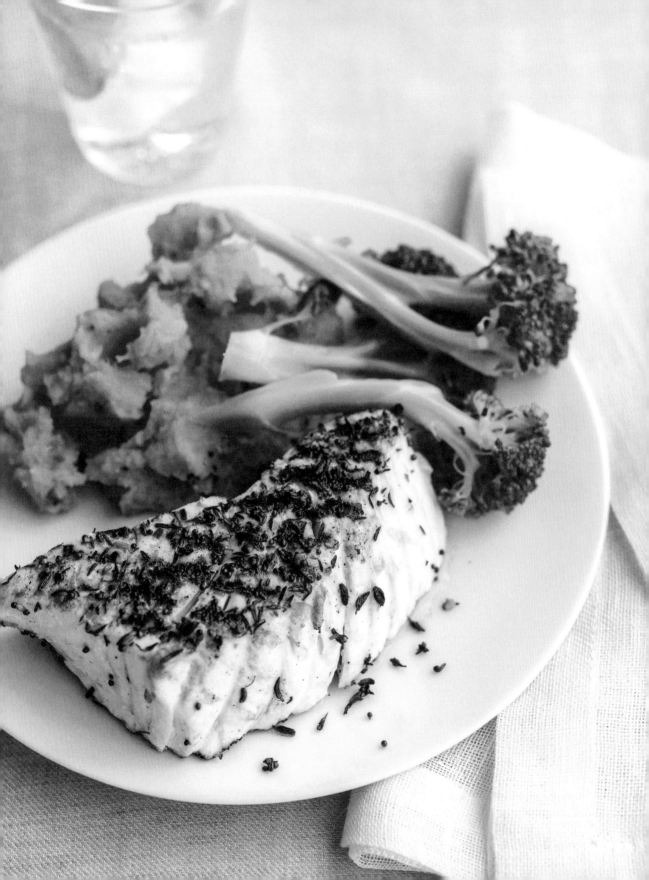

Skewered
SHRIMP

Dill and lemon pair perfectly with shrimp, which we make easy to grill by threading them on skewers with grape tomatoes.

ACTIVE TIME: 25 MINUTES **TOTAL TIME:** 30 MINUTES
MAKES: 8 MAIN-DISH SERVINGS

15 bamboo skewers (10 inches each)

2 lemons, plus additional lemon wedges for garnish

2 tablespoons olive oil

1 large garlic clove, crushed with press

4 tablespoons chopped fresh dill, plus additional sprigs for garnish

½ teaspoon salt

¼ teaspoon ground black pepper

2¼ pounds large shrimp, peeled and deveined

1 pint grape tomatoes

1 Soak skewers in *hot water* for at least 30 minutes. Prepare outdoor grill for direct grilling over medium heat.

2 From lemons, grate 4 teaspoons peel and squeeze 2 tablespoons juice. In large bowl with wire whisk or fork, mix lemon peel and juice, olive oil, garlic, 3 tablespoons chopped dill, salt, and pepper until blended. Add shrimp; toss to coat.

3 Alternately thread shrimp and tomatoes on skewers. Place skewers on hot grill rack. Cook for 4 to 5 minutes or until shrimp are just opaque throughout and tomatoes are slightly charred, turning skewers occasionally.

4 To serve, transfer skewers to platter; sprinkle with remaining 1 tablespoon dill. Garnish with lemon wedges and dill sprigs.

EACH SERVING: ABOUT 175 CALORIES, 26G PROTEIN, 4G CARBOHYDRATE, 6G TOTAL FAT (1G SATURATED), 1G FIBER, 194MG CHOLESTEROL, 340MG SODIUM.

SCALLOP & CHERRY TOMATO
Skewers

Fresh lemon and Dijon mustard give these
grilled skewers their zesty flavor.

ACTIVE TIME: 20 MINUTES   **TOTAL TIME:** 30 MINUTES
MAKES: 4 MAIN-DISH SERVINGS

8   bamboo skewers (8 inches each)

1   lemon

2   tablespoons olive oil

2   tablespoons Dijon mustard

$\frac{1}{8}$ teaspoon salt

24 cherry tomatoes

16 large sea scallops (1¼ pounds total)

1 Soak skewers in *hot water* for at least 30 minutes. Prepare outdoor grill for direct grilling over medium heat.

2 Meanwhile, from lemon, grate 1½ teaspoons peel and squeeze 1 tablespoon juice. In small bowl with wire whisk, mix lemon peel and juice, oil, Dijon, and salt until well blended; set aside.

3 Alternately thread 3 tomatoes and 2 scallops on each skewer, beginning and ending with tomatoes.

4 Brush scallops and tomatoes with half of Dijon mixture. Place skewers on hot grill rack. Cook for 7 to 9 minutes, turning several times. Brush with remaining Dijon mixture, and cook for 5 minutes more or until scallops are just opaque throughout.

EACH SERVING: ABOUT 215 CALORIES, 25G PROTEIN, 9G CARBOHYDRATE, 9G TOTAL FAT (1G SATURATED), 1G FIBER, 47MG CHOLESTEROL, 335MG SODIUM.

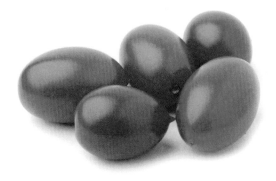

TIP

If you see a white strip (i.e., a muscle) along the short edge of a scallop, we suggest removing it before cooking. While the muscle is perfectly edible, it tends to be the toughest part of an otherwise delicately textured shellfish.

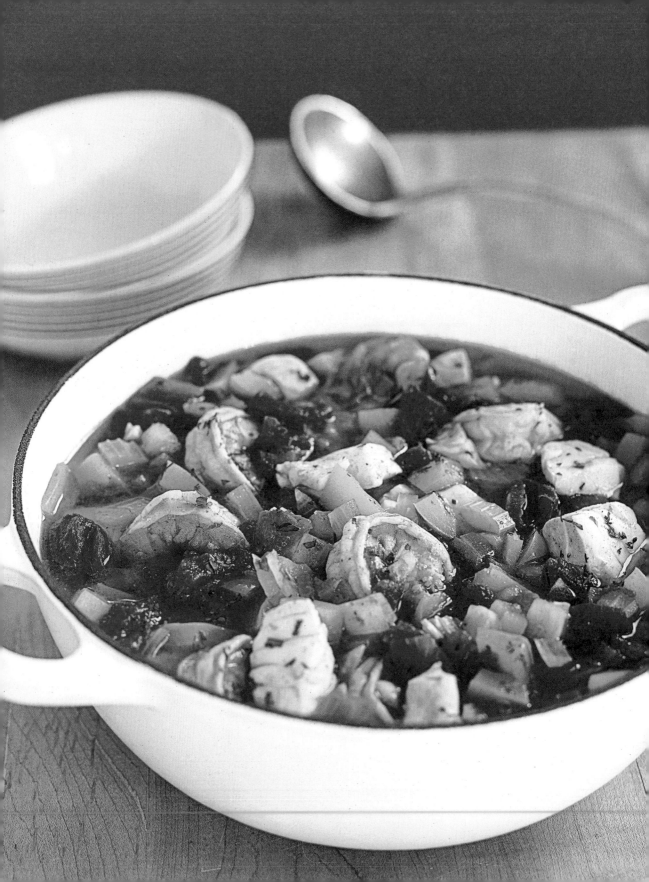

FISHERMAN'S
Stew

This hearty stew is swimming with shrimp
and cod. Feel free to substitute sea scallops
or clams for the shrimp, if you like.

ACTIVE TIME: 15 MINUTES   **TOTAL TIME:** 45 MINUTES
MAKES: 4 MAIN-DISH SERVINGS

1   tablespoon olive oil

1   medium onion, chopped

1   yellow pepper, chopped

1   stalk celery, chopped

2   garlic cloves, crushed with press

1   teaspoon Cajun seasoning

1   can (14½ ounces) diced tomatoes

½   cup dry white wine

½   pound cod fillet, cut into 1-inch chunks

½   pound medium shrimp, peeled and deveined

1 In 4-quart saucepan, heat oil over medium-high heat until hot. Add onion, pepper, and celery and cook, stirring occasionally, for 8 to 10 minutes or until onion is tender and golden. Stir in garlic and Cajun seasoning and cook, stirring, for 1 minute or until fragrant.

2 Add tomatoes, *1 cup water*, and wine; heat to boiling. Reduce heat to medium-low and simmer, covered, for 10 minutes.

3 Stir in cod and shrimp. Cover and simmer for 3 to 4 minutes more or until cod and shrimp are just opaque throughout, gently stirring once.

4 Ladle stew into four large soup bowls.

EACH SERVING: ABOUT 190 CALORIES, 24G PROTEIN, 12G CARBOHYDRATE, 5G TOTAL FAT (1G SATURATED), 2G FIBER, 111MG CHOLESTEROL, 709MG SODIUM.

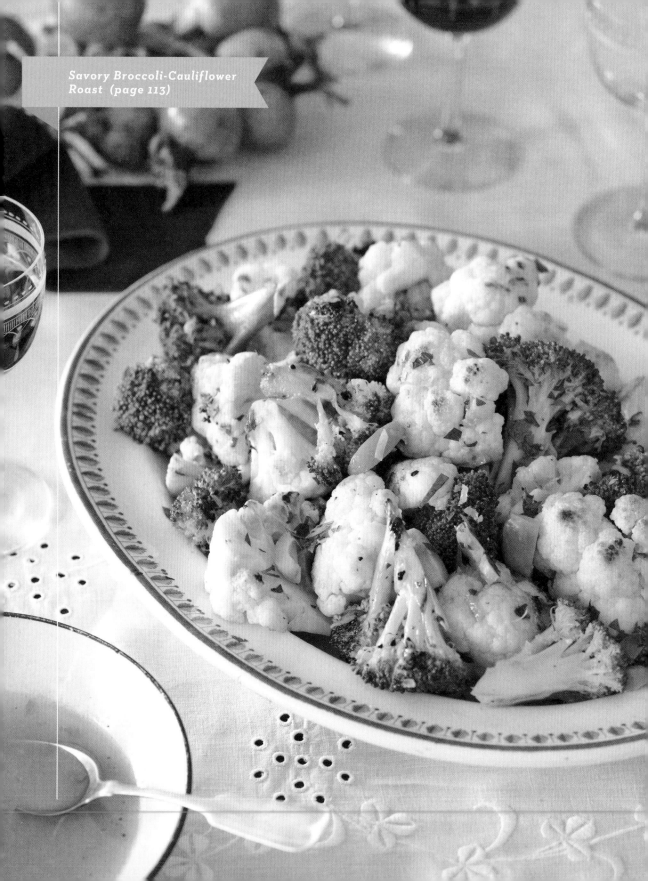

Savory Broccoli-Cauliflower
Roast (page 113)

6 Get Your Fruits & Veggies

No paleo meal would be complete without an ample portion of fresh fruits and vegetables. So we've gathered the best garden-fresh dishes for every season, from Savory Broccoli-Cauliflower Roast and Poached Leeks with Walnut Vinaigrette for winter to springtime Caramelized Carrots, to summery Spiced Ratatouille, to trendy Smoky Paprika Grapes for fall. Plus, if you're looking for a healthy appetizer or snack, our delicious Avocado Pico de Gallo and Kale "Chips" are sure to satisfy your hungry crew.

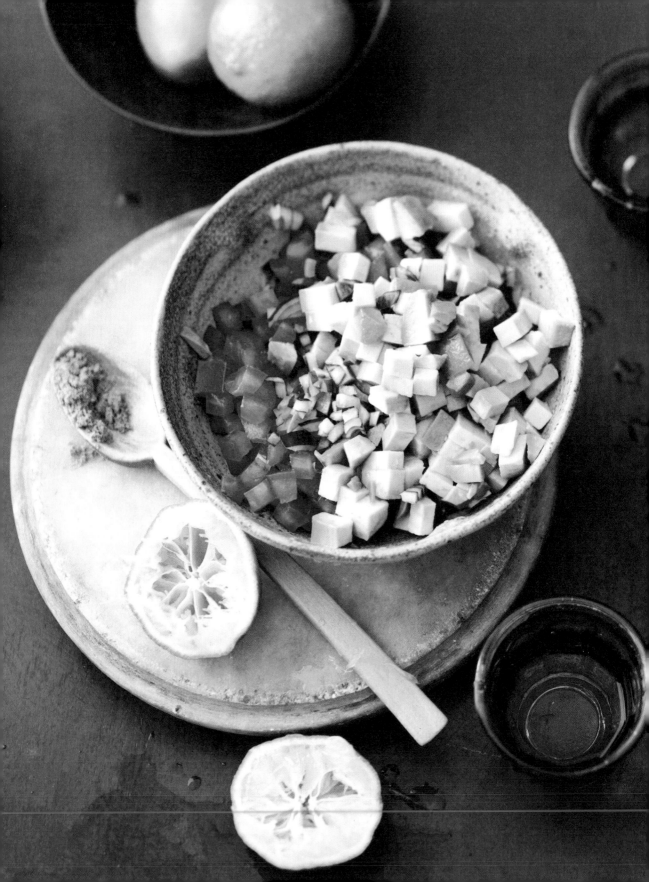

AVOCADO
Pico de Gallo

In Mexico, pico de gallo has the same ingredients as
traditional tomato salsa but with less liquid, so it can be served
not only as an appetizer but as a side dish or salad.
Avocado adds richness and a lovely creamy texture.

TOTAL TIME: 15 MINUTES   **MAKES:** 2¾ CUPS

2   medium ripe avocados, cut into ½-inch chunks

2   plum tomatoes, seeded and coarsely chopped

1   jalapeño chile, chopped

⅓   cup chopped onion

¼   cup loosely packed fresh cilantro leaves, chopped

2   tablespoons fresh lime juice

½   teaspoon kosher salt

Jicama and carrot slices, optional

In medium bowl, combine avocados, tomatoes, jalapeño, onion, cilantro, lime juice, and salt. Store covered in the refrigerator for up to 4 hours. Serve with jicama and carrot slices, if desired.

EACH ¼-CUP SERVING: ABOUT 60 CALORIES, 1G PROTEIN, 4G CARBOHYDRATE, 5G TOTAL FAT (1G SATURATED), 2G FIBER, 0MG CHOLESTEROL, 95MG SODIUM.

TIP

This recipe also makes a great topping for grilled chicken or fish.

KALE "Chips"

Taste the difference! Our DIY kale chips beat any commercial brand that's loaded with salt and are particularly delicious with Red Russian kale, which is sweeter than curly kale.

ACTIVE TIME: 10 MINUTES   **TOTAL TIME:** 25 MINUTES
MAKES: 6 SIDE-DISH SERVINGS (6 CUPS)

1   bunch kale (10 ounces), rinsed and dried well

½   teaspoon kosher salt

1   Preheat oven to 350°F.

2   From kale, remove and discard thick stems and tear leaves into large pieces. Spread leaves in single layer on two large cookie sheets. Spray leaves with nonstick cooking spray to coat lightly; sprinkle with salt.

3   Bake for 12 to 15 minutes or just until kale chips are crisp but not browned. Cool on cookie sheets on wire racks.

EACH SERVING: ABOUT 15 CALORIES, 1G PROTEIN, 3G CARBOHYDRATE, 0G TOTAL FAT, 1G FIBER, 0MG CHOLESTEROL, 175MG SODIUM.

SIMPLE Broccoli Stir-Fry

Tossing and coating broccoli in hot oil before adding water to complete the cooking keeps it beautifully green. For an extra kick of flavor, add chopped fresh ginger or crushed red pepper with the garlic.

ACTIVE TIME: 5 MINUTES   **TOTAL TIME:** 10 MINUTES
MAKES: 6 SIDE-DISH SERVINGS (6 CUPS)

1   bunch broccoli

1   tablespoon olive oil

¼   teaspoon salt

2   garlic cloves, thinly sliced

1   Cut broccoli tops into florets; peel stems and cut into ¼-inch-thick slices.

2   In 12-inch skillet, heat oil over medium-high heat until hot. Add broccoli; sprinkle with salt and cook, stirring constantly, for 1 minute or until well coated and bright green. Add garlic and cook, stirring, for 1 minute or until fragrant.

3   Add ½ cup water; cook, stirring occasionally, for 3 to 5 minutes more or until broccoli is tender-crisp and water evaporates.

EACH SERVING: ABOUT 65 CALORIES, 3G PROTEIN, 6G CARBOHYDRATE, 4G TOTAL FAT (1G SATURATED), 3G FIBER, 0MG CHOLESTEROL, 175MG SODIUM.

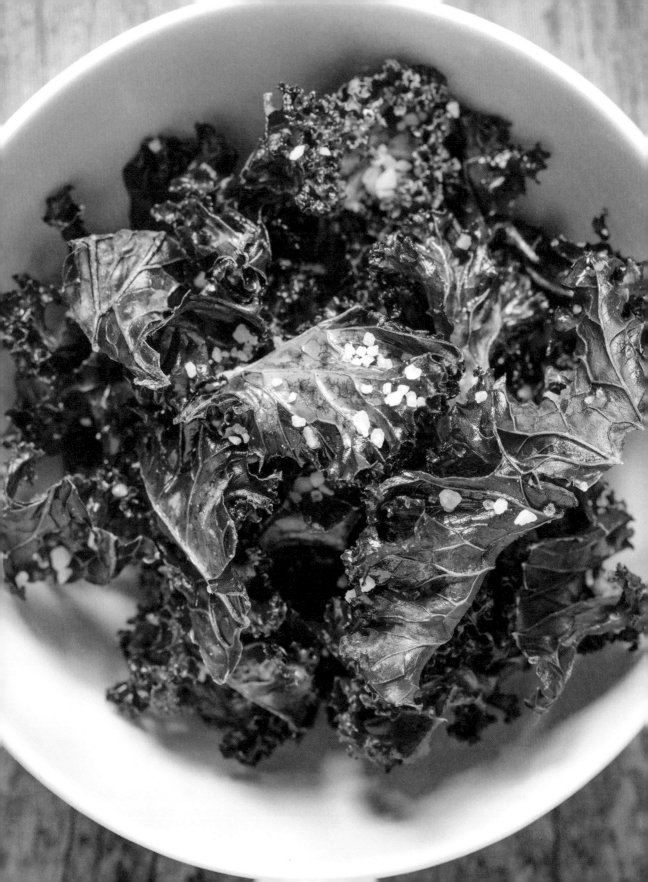

SMOKY PAPRIKA
Grapes

These grilled grapes pair perfectly with our Pork Loin with
Lemon, Thyme & Garlic (page 55) and are
also delicious alongside grilled chicken.

ACTIVE TIME: 5 MINUTES **TOTAL TIME:** 10 MINUTES
MAKES: 4 MAIN-DISH SERVINGS

1 tablespoon olive oil

½ teaspoon smoked paprika

¼ teaspoon salt

⅛ teaspoon cayenne (ground red) pepper

1 large bunch seedless red grapes (1 pound),
separated into smaller clusters but still
on stems

1 Prepare outdoor grill for covered direct
grilling over medium heat.

2 In medium bowl, mix oil, paprika, salt, and
cayenne. Add grapes and toss to coat.

3 Place grapes on hot grill rack. Cover and cook
for 4 to 5 minutes or until grill marks appear,
turning over once.

EACH SERVING: ABOUT 71 CALORIES, 1G PROTEIN,
13G CARBOHYDRATE, 2G TOTAL FAT (0G SATURATED),
1G FIBER, 0MG CHOLESTEROL, 84KMG SODIUM.

TIP
Use scissors to separate the grapes into
small clusters.

SAVORY
Broccoli-Cauliflower Roast

We season this veggie duo with citrus juice and peel, extra-virgin olive oil, chopped green olives, and parsley. For photo, see page 106.

ACTIVE TIME: 15 MINUTES   **TOTAL TIME:** 45 MINUTES
MAKES: 12 SIDE-DISH SERVINGS

4 medium heads broccoli (1½ pounds each), cut into medium florets

5 tablespoons extra-virgin olive oil

Salt and ground black pepper

2 small heads cauliflower (1¼ pounds each), cut into medium florets

1 navel orange

1 lemon

¼ cup pitted green olives, thinly sliced

1 tablespoon fresh flat-leaf parsley leaves, chopped, for garnish

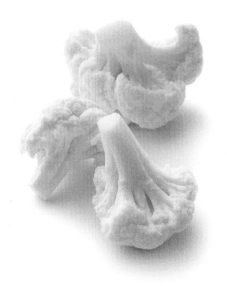

1 Arrange two oven racks in bottom half of oven. Preheat oven to 450°F.

2 On 18" by 12" jelly-roll pan, toss broccoli with 2 tablespoons oil, ¼ teaspoon salt, and ⅛ teaspoon pepper. On another 18" by 12" jelly-roll pan, toss cauliflower with 1 tablespoon oil, ¼ teaspoon salt, and ⅛ teaspoon pepper.

3 Roast for 30 to 35 minutes or until vegetables are browned and just tender, rotating pans between racks halfway through roasting.

4 Meanwhile, from orange, grate ½ teaspoon peel and squeeze ¼ cup juice into medium bowl. Into same bowl, from lemon, grate ¼ teaspoon peel and squeeze 2 tablespoons juice. Whisk in remaining 2 tablespoons oil, ⅛ teaspoon salt, and pinch pepper.

5 Arrange broccoli and cauliflower on serving platter. Scatter olives over vegetables. Whisk dressing again and drizzle all over dish. Garnish with parsley.

EACH SERVING: ABOUT 115 CALORIES, 5G PROTEIN, 12G CARBOHYDRATE, 7G TOTAL FAT (1G SATURATED), 5G FIBER, 0MG CHOLESTEROL, 215MG SODIUM.

GRILLED
Sweet Potatoes

A fragrant spiced oil with paprika, cumin, cinnamon, and pepper gives these sweet spuds their deliciously different flavor.

ACTIVE TIME: 15 MINUTES **TOTAL TIME:** 40 MINUTES
MAKES: 8 SIDE-DISH SERVINGS

2 tablespoons olive oil

1 teaspoon paprika

½ teaspoon ground cumin

½ teaspoon ground cinnamon

½ teaspoon salt

½ teaspoon ground black pepper

3 pounds sweet potatoes

1 Place sweet potatoes in large saucepot; cover with *cold water*. Cover and heat to boiling. Partially uncover. Reduce heat and simmer for 18 minutes or until just tender. Drain; cool slightly. Peel potatoes; cut into ½-inch-thick ovals.

2 Meanwhile, prepare outdoor grill for direct grilling over medium-high heat.

3 In small bowl, combine oil, paprika, cumin, cinnamon, salt, and pepper. Brush large jelly-roll pan with half of spiced oil. Arrange potatoes in pan; brush lightly with more spiced oil.

4 Place potatoes on hot grill rack. Cook for 3 minutes per side or until evenly charred, brushing with remaining spiced oil.

EACH SERVING: ABOUT 133 CALORIES, 2G PROTEIN, 24G CARBOHYDRATE, 4G TOTAL FAT (1G SATURATED), 4G FIBER, 0MG CHOLESTEROL, 159MG SODIUM.

The Paleo Potato: Sweets!

While potatoes are a no-no on the paleo diet (occasionally you can sneak one in), there's one exception: sweet potatoes. An excellent source of vitamin A, good source of vitamin C, and rich in fiber, sweets offer a nutritious, satisfying accompaniment to a host of meals. Plus, they're easy to prepare! Try these basics:

SAUTÉED SWEETS Slice or dice; sauté in olive or coconut oil for about 10 minutes.

QUICK-BOIL SWEETS Combine 1-inch slices and 2 inches boiling water in skillet; cook for about 12 minutes.

MICRO-BAKE SWEETS Microwave whole sweet potatoes for 4 minutes, then bake at 450°F for 5 to 10 minutes.

BROILED SWEETS Cut into 1-inch slices; broil for 10 minutes, turning over once.

RAW SWEETS Grate raw into slaws and salads.

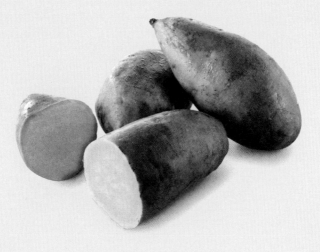

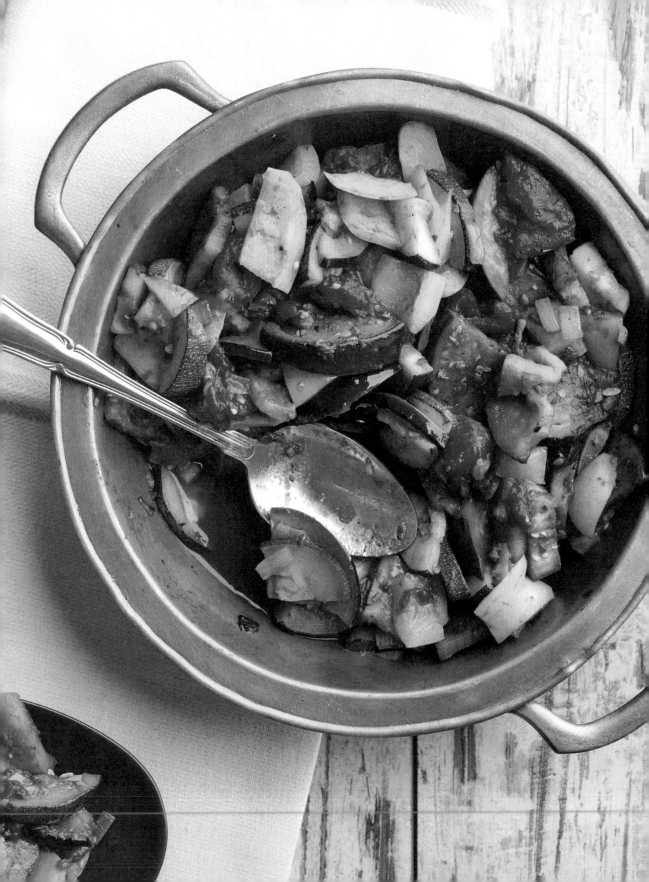

SPICED
Ratatouille

We jazzed up this summer classic with coriander,
crushed red pepper, and cinnamon.
Serve warm, chilled, or at room temperature.

ACTIVE TIME: 20 MINUTES   **TOTAL TIME:** 50 MINUTES PLUS STANDING
MAKES: 4 SIDE-DISH SERVINGS

1   medium eggplant, peeled and cut into 1-inch cubes

¾   teaspoon salt

3   tablespoons olive oil

2   small red peppers, chopped

1   medium onion, finely chopped

3   garlic cloves, chopped

1¼ teaspoons ground coriander

½   teaspoon crushed red pepper

¼   teaspoon ground cinnamon

12 ounces summer squash, chopped

2   medium tomatoes, chopped

2   teaspoons red wine vinegar

¼   teaspoon ground black pepper

1 Sprinkle eggplant with ¼ teaspoon salt. Let stand for 20 minutes; squeeze liquid from eggplant with paper towels.

2 In large saucepot, heat oil over medium-high heat until hot. Add eggplant and cook, stirring, for 5 minutes. With slotted spoon, transfer to bowl.

3 To same pot, add red peppers, onion, garlic, coriander, crushed red pepper, cinnamon, and remaining ½ teaspoon salt. Cook, stirring, for 4 minutes. Stir in squash, tomatoes, and remaining 1 tablespoon oil; cook, stirring, for 10 minutes. Add eggplant. Reduce heat and simmer for 10 minutes or until vegetables are tender. Remove pot from heat; stir in vinegar and black pepper.

EACH SERVING: ABOUT 172 CALORIES, 4G PROTEIN, 18G CARBOHYDRATE, 11G TOTAL FAT (2G SATURATED), 6G FIBER, 0MG CHOLESTEROL, 379MG SODIUM.

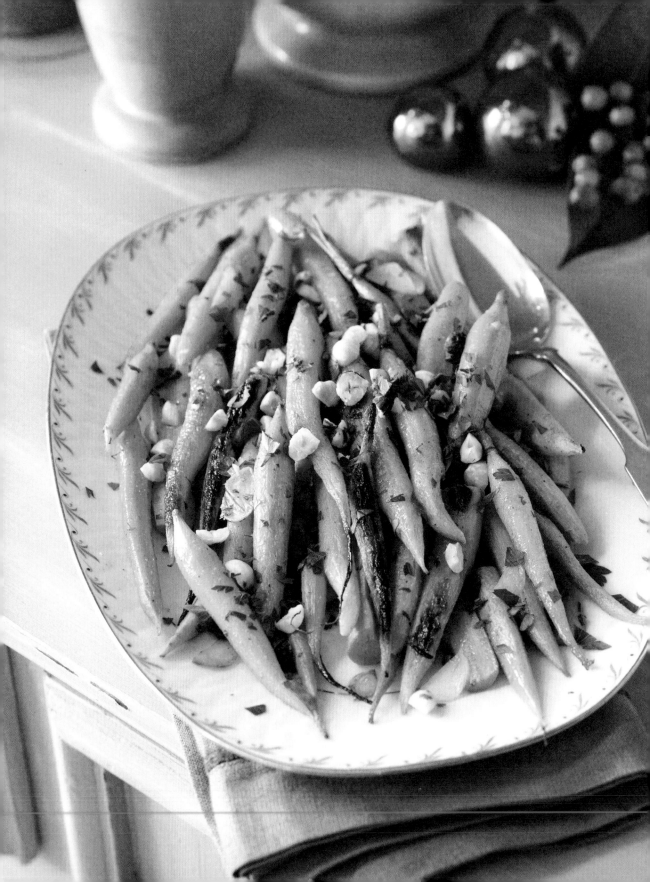

CARAMELIZED
Carrots

Petite-sized carrots tossed with olive oil, garlic, and warm spices are roasted and then sprinkled with chopped toasted hazelnuts.

ACTIVE TIME: 20 MINUTES   **TOTAL TIME:** 45 MINUTES
MAKES: 12 SIDE-DISH SERVINGS

½ cup hazelnuts (filberts)

3 pounds small carrots, peeled

1 garlic clove, very thinly sliced

½ teaspoon ground ginger

½ teaspoon smoked paprika

2 tablespoons plus 1 teaspoon olive oil

½ teaspoon salt

¼ teaspoon ground black pepper

¼ cup packed fresh flat-leaf parsley leaves

1 Preheat oven to 350°F. Place hazelnuts in 18" by 12" jelly-roll pan. Bake for 10 to 12 minutes or until toasted. Wrap hot hazelnuts in clean cloth towel. With hands, roll hazelnuts back and forth to remove skins; discard skins. Let toasted hazelnuts cool completely; set aside.

2 In same pan, toss carrots with garlic, ginger, paprika, 2 tablespoons oil, salt, and pepper. Cover pan tightly with foil and roast for 30 minutes. Uncover and roast for 20 to 25 minutes more or until carrots are tender.

3 Meanwhile, in food processor with knife blade attached, pulse hazelnuts and parsley until coarsely chopped; set hazelnut mixture aside.

4 Remove carrots from oven and drizzle with remaining 1 teaspoon oil, tossing well to coat. Transfer carrots to large serving dish or platter and sprinkle with hazelnut mixture.

EACH SERVING: ABOUT 100 CALORIES, 2G PROTEIN, 11G CARBOHYDRATE, 6G TOTAL FAT (1G SATURATED), 4G FIBER, 0MG CHOLESTEROL, 170MG SODIUM.

TIP

This recipe is best with small carrots (not pre-packed baby carrots), or you can use large carrots cut in quarters lengthwise, then halved.

SAUTÉED SWISS CHARD
with Golden Raisins & Capers

Naturally sweet raisins and piquant capers enliven
the rich, earthy flavor of Swiss chard.

ACTIVE TIME: 30 MINUTES **TOTAL TIME:** 50 MINUTES
MAKES: 4 SIDE-DISH SERVINGS

2   pounds Swiss chard

1   tablespoon olive oil

1   small onion, chopped

⅓   cup golden raisins

2   tablespoons capers, drained

Chopped walnuts, for garnish (optional)

1 Trim tough stem ends from Swiss chard. Cut stems crosswise into 1-inch pieces; cut leaves into 2-inch pieces, keeping stems and leaves separate.

2 In 12-inch nonstick skillet, heat oil over medium-high heat until hot. Add onion and cook, stirring occasionally, for about 4 minutes or until onion begins to brown. Add chard stems; cover and cook, stirring occasionally, for 5 to 7 minutes or until tender. Stir in raisins.

3 Add leaves to stems in batches, covering skillet after each batch; cook, stirring often, for 7 to 10 minutes or until leaves are tender and wilted. Remove from heat; stir in capers. Garnish with walnuts, if desired.

EACH SERVING: ABOUT 120 CALORIES, 4G PROTEIN, 20G CARBOHYDRATE, 4G TOTAL FAT (1G SATURATED), 5G FIBER, 0MG CHOLESTEROL, 555MG SODIUM.

TIP

Substitute kale or peppery mustard greens for the chard, if you wish.

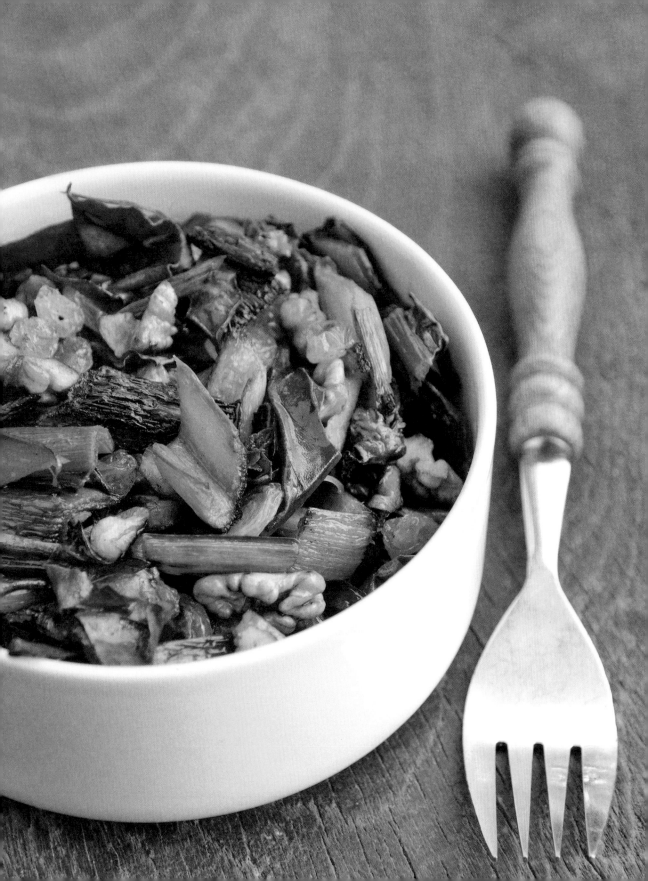

VEGETABLE
Kebabs

These simple kebabs of grilled bell peppers and sweet onions make the perfect summer side for grilled meats, like our Butterflied Leg of Lamb with Mint Pesto (page 64).

ACTIVE TIME: 20 MINUTES   **TOTAL TIME:** 30 MINUTES
MAKES: 6 SIDE-DISH SERVINGS

8 wooden skewers (8 inches each)

4 medium orange, red, and/or yellow peppers

2 medium sweet onions

2 tablespoons olive or avocado oil

½ teaspoon salt

¼ teaspoon coarsely ground black pepper

1 Soak skewers in *hot water* for at least 30 minutes. Prepare outdoor grill for direct covered grilling over medium heat.

2 Cut peppers into 1-inch pieces. Cut onions into 8 wedges each, then cut each wedge crosswise in half. Alternately thread peppers and onions onto skewers; place in jelly-roll pan. Brush vegetables with oil and sprinkle with salt and pepper.

3 Place kebabs on hot grill rack. Cover and cook for 8 to 9 minutes or until vegetables are lightly charred and tender, turning occasionally.

....

EACH SERVING: ABOUT 65 CALORIES, 1G PROTEIN, 8G CARBOHYDRATE, 4G TOTAL FAT (1G SATURATED), 2G FIBER, 0MG CHOLESTEROL, 150MG SODIUM.

POACHED LEEKS WITH
Walnut Vinaigrette

Chopped walnuts and a delicate vinaigrette
with walnut oil, Champagne vinegar, and fresh
rosemary give this French classic a modern twist.

ACTIVE TIME: 20 MINUTES **TOTAL TIME:** 35 MINUTES
MAKES: 4 SIDE-DISH SERVINGS

1¼ teaspoons salt

8 small leeks (about 3 pounds total)

½ cup walnuts, coarsely chopped

1 teaspoon finely chopped fresh rosemary
leaves

¼ cup walnut oil

2 tablespoons Champagne vinegar

2 tablespoons chopped fresh parsley

¼ teaspoon ground black pepper

1 Heat large pot of *water* and 1 teaspoon salt to boiling over high heat.

2 Meanwhile, trim root and dark-green tops from leeks. Discard tough outer leaves. Make lengthwise slit in each leek, being careful not to cut all the way through. Carefully rinse leeks in large bowl of *cold water*, swishing to remove sand; transfer leeks to colander, leaving sand in bowl. Repeat several times, using fresh water. Drain well.

3 Fill large bowl with *ice water* and set aside. Add leeks to boiling water and cook for 7 minutes or until easily pierced with knife. Drain leeks and transfer to bowl of ice water. Drain again and pat dry with paper towels. Transfer leeks to serving dish.

4 In small skillet, cook walnuts and rosemary over medium heat, stirring occasionally, for about 5 minutes or until golden and fragrant.

5 In small bowl with wire whisk, mix vinegar, parsley, remaining ¼ teaspoon salt, and pepper until well blended. Spoon dressing over leeks and sprinkle with walnut mixture.

EACH SERVING: ABOUT 315 CALORIES, 5G PROTEIN, 23G CARBOHYDRATE, 24G TOTAL FAT (2G SATURATED), 4G FIBER, 0MG CHOLESTEROL, 205MG SODIUM.

Index

Note: Page numbers in *italics* indicate photos on pages separate from recipes.

Photography Credits

Cover: Mike Garten; back cover: © Kate Mathis

Alamy: © Funky Stock—Paul Williams: 115

© James Baigre: 19, 54, 65, 79, 101

Depositphotos: ©Nik_merkulov: 9; © paulistano: 43

© Tara Donne: 95

Chris Eckert/Studio D: 7

Mike Garten: 2, 6, 36, 53, 96

Getty Images: © Amana Productions, Inc.: 34 (oak leaf); © Rita Maas: 63; Maximilian Stock Ltd.: 34 (lolla rossa); Tony Robins: 17; © Westend61: 15

iStock: © anna1311: 93; © Floortje: 113; © Givaga: 68; © Gabor Izso: 103; © macida: 83; © OliverChilds: 29; © john shepherd: 34 (mizuna); © Alasdair Thomson: 34 (frisee);

© Francis Janisch: 104

© Yunhee Kim: 106

© Kate Mathis: 22, 31, 38, 41, 49, 61, 71, 84, 89, 92, 99, 118

© Con Poulos: 72, 77

© David Prince: 74

Emily Kate Roemer/Studio D: 12, 66

© Kate Sears: 58, 81

Shutterstock: © Madlen: 34; © Pinkyone: 111

StockFood: © Grafe & Unzer: 108; © Meike Bergmann: 116

Stocksy: © Harald Walker: 121

© Anna Williams: 26, 33, 44

Metric Conversion Charts

The recipes that appear in this cookbook use the standard United States method for measuring liquid and dry or solid ingredients (teaspoons, tablespoons, and cups). The information on this chart is provided to help cooks outside the U.S. successfully use these recipes. All equivalents are approximate.

METRIC EQUIVALENTS FOR DIFFERENT TYPES OF INGREDIENTS

STANDARD CUP	FINE POWDER (e.g. flour)	GRAIN (e.g. rice)	GRANULAR (e.g. sugar)	LIQUID SOLIDS (e.g. butter)	LIQUID (e.g. milk)
¾	105 g	113 g	143 g	150 g	180 ml
⅔	93 g	100 g	125 g	133 g	160 ml
½	70 g	75 g	95 g	100 g	120 ml
⅓	47 g	50 g	63 g	67 g	80 ml
¼	35 g	38 g	48 g	50 g	60 ml
⅛	18 g	19 g	24 g	25 g	30 ml

USEFUL EQUIVALENTS FOR LIQUID INGREDIENTS BY VOLUME

¼ tsp	=						1 ml	
½ tsp	=						2 ml	
1 tsp	=						5 ml	
3 tsp	=	1 tbls	=		½ fl oz	=	15 ml	
		2 tbls	=	⅛ cup	=	1 fl oz	=	30 ml
		4 tbls	=	¼ cup	=	2 fl oz	=	60 ml
		5⅓ tbls	=	⅓ cup	=	3 fl oz	=	80 ml
		8 tbls	=	½ cup	=	4 fl oz	=	120 ml
		10⅔ tbls	=	⅔ cup	=	5 fl oz	=	160 ml
		12 tbls	=	¾ cup	=	6 fl oz	=	180 ml
		16 tbls	=	1 cup	=	8 fl oz	=	240 ml
		1 pt	=	2 cups	=	16 fl oz	=	480 ml
		1 qt	=	4 cups	=	32 fl oz	=	960 ml
						33 fl oz	=	1000 ml = 1 L

USEFUL EQUIVALENTS FOR DRY INGREDIENTS BY WEIGHT

(To convert ounces to grams, multiply the number of ounces by 30.)

1 oz	=	¹⁄₁₆ lb	=	30 g
4 oz	=	¼ lb	=	120 g
8 oz	=	½ lb	=	240 g
12 oz	=	¾ lb	=	360 g
16 oz	=	1 lb	=	480 g

USEFUL EQUIVALENTS FOR COOKING/OVEN TEMPERATURES

	Fahrenheit	Celsius	Gas Mark
Freeze Water	32° F	0° C	
Room Temperature	68° F	20° C	
Boil Water	212° F	100° C	
Bake	325° F	160° C	3
	350° F	180° C	4
	375° F	190° C	5
	400° F	200° C	6
	425° F	220° C	7
	450° F	230° C	8
Broil			Grill

USEFUL EQUIVALENTS LENGTH

(To convert inches to centimeters, multiply the number of inches by 2.5.)

1 in	=			2.5 cm		
6 in	=	½ ft	=	15 cm		
12 in	=	1 ft	=	30 cm		
36 in	=	3 ft	= 1 yd	=	90 cm	
40 in	=			100 cm	=	1 m

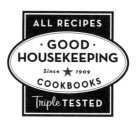

The Good Housekeeping
Triple-Test Promise

At *Good Housekeeping*, we want to make sure that every recipe we print works in any oven, with any brand of ingredient, no matter what. That's why, in our test kitchens at the **Good Housekeeping Research Institute**, we go all out: We test each recipe at least three times—and, often, several more times after that.

When a recipe is first developed, one member of our team prepares the dish, and we judge it on these criteria: It must be **delicious**, **family-friendly**, **healthy**, and **easy to make**.

1 The recipe is then tested several more times to fine-tune the flavor and ease of preparation, always by the same team member, using the same equipment.

2 Next, another team member follows the recipe as written, **varying the brands of ingredients** and **kinds of equipment**. Even the types of stoves we use are changed.

3 A third team member repeats the whole process **using yet another set of equipment** and **alternative ingredients**. By the time the recipes appear on these pages, they are guaranteed to work in any kitchen, including yours. **We promise**.